Interpreting Statistical Findings
A guide for health professionals and students

Jan Walker and Palo Almond

Open University Press

Open University Press
McGraw-Hill Education
McGraw-Hill House
Shoppenhangers Road
Maidenhead
Berkshire
England
SL6 2QL

email: enquiries@openup.co.uk
world wide web: www.openup.co.uk

and Two Penn Plaza, New York, NY 10121-2289, USA

First published 2010

A catalogue record of this book is available from the British Library

ISBN-13: 978-0-33-523597-1 (pb) 978-0-33-523596-4 (hb)
ISBN-10: 0-33-523597-2 (pb) 0-33-523596-4 (hb)

Library of Congress Cataloging-in-Publication Data
CIP data applied for

Typeset by Graphicraft Limited, Hong Kong
Printed in the UK by Bell & Bain Ltd., Glasgow

Fictitious names of companies, products, people, characters and/or data that may
be used herein (in case studies or in examples) are not intended to represent any
real individual, company, product or event.

Mixed Sources
Product group from well-managed
forests and other controlled sources
www.fsc.org   Cert no. TT-COC-002769
© 1996 Forest Stewardship Council

FSC

The **McGraw·Hill** Companies

Contents

List of Figures

List of Tables

Acknowledgements

We would like to thank the following whose constructive feedback shaped the development of this book: Beverley French, who conducted a thorough review of the content and presentation following submission of the first complete draft; Stephanie Wheeler, who thoughtfully reviewed much of the final content; and the various undergraduate and postgraduate, public health, nursing and medical students who commented on early chapter drafts – Amanda Cain, Laura Caddis, Dharam Dickinson, Karin Downer, Donna Forbes, Jane Levers and Dianne Rogers.

Praise for this book

"The authors of this text have gone out of their way to make statistics accessible, and to structure learning into progressive stages. They have also not taken anything for granted in terms of understanding, and have included an explanation of even very basic concepts. Particularly useful is showing how the statistics in the original paper are arrived at, and highlighting salient points in extracts from tables of the original study.

This book would reward careful study, and provide excellent preparation for practitioners undertaking courses in evidence-based practice or research."

Dr Beverley French, Senior Research Fellow,
University of Central Lancashire, UK

Introduction

This book is aimed primarily at honours undergraduate and postgraduate students, working in health and social care and conducting a critical review of research evidence for practice or for a dissertation.

Few people working in these fields, even some researchers, have sufficient knowledge and confidence to critique the results section of a quantitative study. We know that many students base their conclusions on the researchers' own interpretation of the data. However, in preparing this book we have identified many anomalies in peer-reviewed research and want to share ways of spotting such problems. It requires basic knowledge of statistical concepts and some interesting detective work.

The book is presented in the form of a manual that provides basic knowledge, review templates and a rough guide to statistical information. Students who reviewed early content advised us that it is sometimes necessary to read parts of it several times in order to understand it properly. Be reassured that it has taken us years to understand some aspects ourselves and we are still learning!

How to use this book

We have divided the content into four parts. **Part 1** contains worked examples of the two main types of research method used in health care: the randomised controlled trial (Chapter 1) and the health survey (Chapter 2). These provide exemplars and templates for statistical review. They will also help you to identify gaps in your knowledge to which you should find answers in Parts 2 and 3.

Part 2 contains nine chapters, each of which addresses a basic statistical concept. Examples are used throughout to illustrate each concept and explain its influence on the research results.

Part 3 focuses on common statistical tests and their applications. Each chapter explains the type of test, the assumptions on which it is based, and the presentation and interpretation of the results.

Throughout Parts 1–3, examples are displayed in text boxes.

Part 4 provides a series of 'quick reference guides' for those who wish to refresh their memories, look up a specific term or check out a result using a statistical table, while conducting their own review.

We offer some suggestions for further reading. Internet sites are particularly helpful, but are subject to change. Of these, university sites are most reliable (look for those ending in '.ac.uk' or '.edu'), some even provide lecture notes. Some commercial research sites provide useful free information for students. There is some sound information on *Wikipedia*, though we spotted one or two inaccuracies which we regret we failed to stop and correct.

PART 1
WORKED EXAMPLES

This part of the book consists of two chapters that illustrate statistical review for two research methodologies: the randomised controlled trial (Chapter 1) and the health survey (Chapter 2). Each chapter uses a single article to explain aspects of statistical relevance. These were selected arbitrarily from peer-reviewed journals. The subject matter is unlikely to be relevant to practice for most readers, but our aim is to provide transferable knowledge about the process of statistical appraisal.

If you are using these chapters to help you review a paper of your own, we provide review notes to assist, so keep pen and paper to hand.

It is not necessary to have access to the selected papers, but those who choose to will find we have used only extracts and have sometimes adapted material to illustrate key points. We include brief descriptions of statistical terms, but you may need to refer to Parts 2 and 3 for more detailed explanations.

1 The Randomised Controlled Trial

Introduction

The randomised controlled trial (RCT), or clinical trial, is regarded within medical science as the 'gold standard' research methodology for testing the effectiveness of a new or experimental treatment. Key features include:

1. Justified reasons for predicting that the experimental intervention is likely to be as effective as the current best treatment or management, if not more so.
2. A standardised experimental intervention.
3. A control group that receives a comparable intervention in the form of placebo or current best practice.
4. A sample that is representative of the target population and clearly defined by inclusion and exclusion criteria.
5. A sample size sufficiently large to detect a statistically significant difference, if there is one to be found.
6. A set of valid, reliable and sensitive outcome measures.
7. Baseline and follow-up measurements taken over an adequate time scale.
8. Randomised allocation to either the experimental or the control intervention(s).
9. Preferably double blind treatment administration in which neither the patient nor the researcher nor the administering clinician is aware which treatment the patient is receiving.
10. Statistical tests, appropriate to the type and distribution of data, which test the effectiveness of the intervention.

Each of these features can affect the statistical results or their interpretation.

In this chapter we review the following public health study to illustrate each point, and you will find these illustrations in boxes throughout the chapter.

> **Logan et al. (2004)**
> Logan, P.A., Gladman, J.R.F., Avery, A., Walker, M.F., Dyas, J. and Groom, L. (2004) Randomised controlled trial of an occupational therapy to increase outdoor mobility after stroke. *British Medical Journal*, 329: 1372–1375.

Research questions and hypotheses

In an RCT, the research question focuses on whether or not a new treatment (the experimental intervention) will be more effective than either a placebo or current best practice (the control intervention) in producing certain outcomes.

> **Logan et al. (2004)**
> Logan et al. set out to study if the introduction of a brief occupational therapy (OT) intervention would improve outdoor mobility and quality of life for post-stroke patients in care homes. This was compared to current practice which involved a single assessment visit.

The primary purpose of the hypotheses is to determine which outcome variables need to be measured and tested. They may be stated explicitly or should be easily deduced from the aim or research question.

> **Logan et al. (2004)**
> The hypotheses can be deduced as stating that post-stroke patients receiving the new goal-based OT intervention (the experimental intervention) may demonstrate greater improvements in outdoor mobility and quality of life than those receiving routine OT intervention (the control intervention).
>   Thus the outcome variables in this study will be measures of outdoor mobility and quality of life.

The language used to state the hypotheses reflects the degree of certainty with which the outcome can be predicted, based on research evidence presented in the introduction. This in turn determines the test of probability applied to the statistical results (see Chapter 9):

- A strong body of evidence leads the researcher to predict that the new intervention *will* improve outcomes when compared to a suitable control intervention. This normally justifies using a directional test of probability (known as a one-tailed test) to interpret the statistical results.

- Lack of pre-existing evidence leads the researcher to a tentative prediction that the new intervention *may* (or may not) lead to improved outcomes. In this case a non-directional test of probability (known as a two-tailed test) should be used.

As you will see later, the direction of the hypothesis affects the sample size and statistical significance of the study results.

Researchers are usually convinced that the new intervention will prove efficacious. But from an ethical perspective, there must be sufficient justification for doing an RCT but no conclusive evidence that the intervention will be effective for the target population. This is termed 'equipoise'.[1] Therefore, the reviewer should expect all clinical trials to apply a non-directional (two-tailed) test of probability to their results.

---

1 It would be unethical to allocate people to a control group denied a treatment known to be effective.

> **Logan et al. (2004)**
> The objective was to establish *whether* those receiving the OT intervention would benefit. Therefore, we should expect the statistical tests to be interpreted using non-directional (two-tailed) tests of probability.

Review notes:
Make a note of all outcomes predicted by the hypotheses (Chapter 10 gives a suggestion for setting up a recording sheet).
Check that the predicted outcome reflects equipoise.
Remember to check the planned data analysis and results to ensure that a non-directional (two-tailed) test of probability was applied to the statistical analysis.

Standardised experimental and control interventions

Both the experimental and control interventions should be clearly described so that potential sources of treatment bias can be identified. The experimental intervention must be standardised and its active ingredients clearly identified so that replication is possible. The control intervention should control for the effects of such factors as:

- the placebo effect;
- additional attention from being in a study (commonly known as the Hawthorne effect);
- healing and other changes attributable to natural processes over time (known as 'regression towards the mean').

> **Logan et al. (2004)**
> The experimental intervention consisted of a standardised assessment visit followed by up to seven goal-based treatment sessions over 3 months.
> The control intervention consisted of the standardised OT assessment visit, including advice and information, followed by usual care.
> You might note that:
>
> - the intervention group gained more visits than the control group, which means that the control intervention is not comparable in terms of the amount of professional attention received;
> - the intervention was not standardised in terms of content or time.
>
> It is important to consider if these could bias the study results.

Review notes:
Are the interventions standardised and described in detail?
Is the control intervention comparable with the experimental intervention?

A representative sample of adequate size

Factors to consider include:

- inclusion and exclusion criteria;
- sampling procedure;
- demographic and other local contextual factors;
- sample size;
- recruitment process.

Inclusion and exclusion criteria

These define the target population and are usually stated in the Method section, under the heading of 'sample' or 'participants'.

> **Logan et al. (2004)**
> The Method section states that the sample consisted of
>
> *'patients with a clinical diagnosis of stroke in the previous 36 months from general practice registers and other sources in the community. We included people in care homes.' (p. 1372)*

Logan et al. give no specific inclusion or exclusion criteria other than stroke duration. This implies the findings should generalize to all patients who have had a stroke within the last 36 months, regardless of stroke duration or severity or previous general health.

As a practitioner, you might question if recruits who had a stroke over a year ago are likely to achieve similar outcomes to those whose stroke was more recent; or if it was logical to include those with pre-existing illnesses or disabilities.

Review notes:
Make a list of the inclusion and exclusion criteria and compare these to patients or clients whom you know to be members of the same target population. Are the criteria clearly stated? Are any important subgroups of individuals excluded or problematic ones included?

The sampling procedure

The study findings only generalise to the target population if the sample is representative of all those who meet the inclusion and exclusion criteria. Multi-centre RCTs achieve this by including a large number of patients from different locations. But most small studies are based on a convenience sample of patients from one or two localities, which means that the outcomes may be subject to local environmental, cultural and socio-economic sources of bias.

> **Logan et al. (2004)**
> This study focused on a convenience sample of patients in one locality which, according to the researchers' address, would appear to be the Trent region of the UK. The reviewer should consider if this region is likely to have particular health needs.

Tables of demographic and baseline data in the Results section may provide clues to sampling bias. Use your professional knowledge and experience of working with similar population groups to inform your judgement.

> **Logan et al. (2004)**
> Table 1 of the Results gives details of male/female balance, age distribution (but not age range), months since stroke, residential status and mobility at the start of the study, which provide useful comparisons with post-stroke patients elsewhere.

Review notes:
Look at the list of inclusion and exclusion criteria. Do they seem comprehensive?
Is there any evidence that the participants in this study might be different from those in other localities?
Is it possible that the local context of care might have influenced the outcomes of the study?

Sample size

The sample size (see Chapter 8) for an RCT must be 'powered' (calculated as adequate) to detect a statistically significant improvement in the intervention group when compared to the control group, assuming there is an improvement to be found. If not, the study is susceptible to Type II error (Type II error is the failure to find a significant outcome when there really is one).

Power calculation is usually undertaken by a statistician, or by using a web-based tool. It is based on the following criteria, which should be applied to each principal outcome measure:

- **effect size**, based on the predicted level of improvement and standard deviation for each measure;
- **significance level**;
- **test of probability** (one-tailed or two-tailed);
- **statistical power**;
- **attrition**.

You should find these details in the Method section, under a heading that includes 'Analysis'. We briefly consider each aspect below.

Logan et al. (2004)
Details of the sample size calculation are given in a section labelled 'statistical analysis':

'In the absence of pilot data for our principal outcome measure, we estimated that we needed a sample size of 200 to detect a three point difference in the scores on the Nottingham activities of daily living scale ($\alpha = 0.05$, power 80%, and standard deviation 5).' (p. 1373)

Clinical effect

Clinical effect is measured by the number of scale points needed to produce a clinically meaningful improvement.

Logan et al. (2004)
Power calculation was based on a mean three-point difference in the Nottingham Extended Activities of Daily Living (EADL) Scale, which is judged to be clinically important. This raises some questions for the reviewer:

1. Does a three-point improvement really represent a clinically relevant outcome for this target population?
Logan et al. fail to justify this level of outcome, so we did our own detective work. Their results section showed that the EADL was measured using a 0–66 point scale. Using Google Scholar with search terms: 'Nottingham Extended Activities of Daily Living', 'stroke' and 'effect', we found that Gilbertson et al. (2000) set a standard 9 points for improvement on the same scale.

2. Does the sample size calculation based on the EADL apply to the other outcome measures used?
Not necessarily. The primary outcome measures were 'gets out of the house as much as wants (yes/no)' and 'number of outdoor journeys taken in the last month'. No existing or pilot data were available for these variables, so no power calculations were included.

Effect size

Some researchers base their sample size on a standardised measure of effect, known as 'effect size', which is generally interpreted (from Cohen 1988) as:

≥0.8	large
0.5–0.8	moderate
0.2–0.5	small.

Anything smaller is trivial. Most researchers would aim for a moderate effect size of at least 0.5.

Assuming that the data conform to the normal distribution and the clinical effect and standard deviation (see Chapter 4) for the measure are known:

$$\text{effect size} = \frac{\text{clinical effect}}{\text{standard deviation (sd)}}.$$

For the Logan et al. data, the clinical effect is 3 EADL scale points and the standard deviation is 5, so

$$\text{effect size} = \frac{3}{5} = 0.6.$$

This would be considered adequate.

Review note:
Look for evidence that the effect size used in the power calculation was based on a realistic assumption about the clinical effect and standard deviation for the primary outcome measure(s).

Significance level

The significance level (also known as alpha, α) is the level of probability that defines the threshold for a statistically significant outcome (see Chapter 9).

The default significance level used in research is $\alpha = 0.05$ (i.e. $p \leq 0.05$). This implies that there is a probability of 0.05 or less that there is *no* effect (the null hypothesis).[2]

Alpha may be set at a more stringent level if the risk of adverse events is high. Where a large number of statistical comparisons are planned, the Bonferroni correction (see Chapter 9) should be applied to identify the level of alpha necessary to avoid Type I error (false significant results). Smaller values of α require a larger sample size to achieve statistical significance.

> **Logan et al. (2004)**
> The significance level used was $\alpha = 0.05$ ($p \leq 0.05$). This seems just about justifiable, given the number of statistical comparisons made (18 in all).

Review note:
Remember to check if the significance level seems appropriate, given the number of statistical tests reported in the Results section.

---

2 Statistical tests all test the null hypothesis, hence smaller values of p indicate a higher level of statistical significance.

Test of probability

A non-directional (two-tailed) test of probability (see Chapter 9) requires a larger sample size to achieve a statistically significant result using the same data, when compared to a directional (one-tailed) test. This can tempt researchers to apply one-tailed tests inappropriately.

> **Logan et al. (2004)**
> Logan et al. applied a non-directional test of probability, in line with their hypothesis.

Review note:
Remember to check that the correct test of probability is applied to the research findings.

Statistical power

This refers to the level of statistical accuracy required (no statistical test is ever 100% accurate). A power of 80%, as used by Logan et al., is the minimum standard of accuracy used in a clinical trial. Sometimes 90% power is used in drug trials where there is a high risk of adverse events; this requires a much larger sample size.

Review note:
Check that the researchers stated the level of statistical power used in their power calculation.

Attrition

When calculating sample size, adequate allowance should be made for attrition (drop-outs) and missing data: 15% is recommended as a minimum.

Actual levels of attrition are usually found in a flow diagram of progress through the study (see Figure 1.1).

Table 1.1 Relationship between attrition and systematic bias

Losses not associated with systematic bias	Losses associated with systematic bias
Unrelated illness or death	Acceptability of the intervention
Family illness or problems	Adverse side-effects
Relocation/job change	Acceptability of the outcome

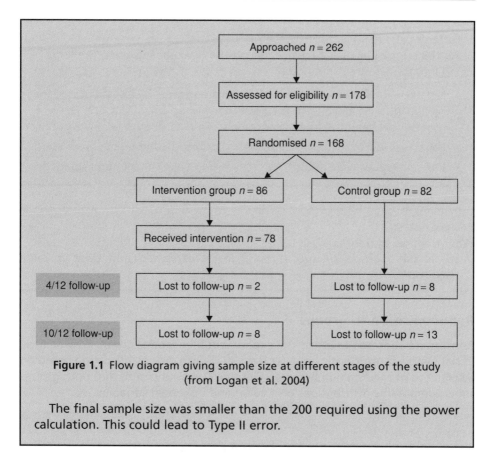

Figure 1.1 Flow diagram giving sample size at different stages of the study (from Logan et al. 2004)

The final sample size was smaller than the 200 required using the power calculation. This could lead to Type II error.

Imbalance in attrition levels between the groups could indicate systematic bias (see Table 1.1).

Review notes:
Is there any evidence of unequal or unreasonable attrition rates? Use clinical knowledge, experience and 'common sense' to speculate about discrepancies that might be associated with any systematic bias in outcomes.
Do the researchers offer adequate explanations for any discrepancies?

It is usual to compensate for imbalance in attrition using 'intention to treat' analysis.

Intention to treat analysis

This involves allocating an outcome score to each lost participant 'as if' they had completed the study, usually by recording no change from baseline.

> **Logan et al. (2004)**
> All 168 original recruits were included in the final analysis using the follow-ing intention-to-treat methods:
>
> - For the main outcome measure, the 'worst outcome' [*sic*] was allocated for participants who had died by the point of follow-up assessment. [We presume that this refers to the lowest outcome score recorded on each measure.]
> - For others lost to follow-up, baseline or last recorded responses were used.
> - Baseline values were substituted for missing values in all other analyses.

Review notes:
Was intention to treat analysis used?
If so, is the method of substitution clearly explained and does it seem reasonable?

Randomisation to groups

Recruits are allocated to either the experimental or control group. Provided the initial sample is sufficiently large (at least 30 in each group), allocation based on a sequence of random numbers (see Chapter 7) should ensure that both groups show comparable distributions on known and unknown variables.

> **Logan et al. (2004)**
> A computer-generated random sequence was used, stratified by age ($\leq$65 and >65) and self-report of dependency on travel (three categories: house-bound, accompanied or independent travel).

The original sample size of 168 was large enough to allow for successful randomisation into two groups. The researchers fail to justify stratification, but it was probably to ensure a balance of small subgroups (see Chapter 7).

Review notes:
Are the authors clear about the method of randomisation used and are there any reasons to doubt its effectiveness?
Check demographic and baseline data for significant group differences that indicate failure of randomisation.

Valid, reliable and sensitive outcome measures

The success of a clinical trial depends on a set of valid and reliable out-come measures that are sufficiently sensitive to detect a clinically relevant and statistically significant group difference. Validity implies that it measures only the outcome it is intended to measure; reliability means that it produces the same measurement consistently when used under the same condition (see Chapter 6 for detailed explanation). The measures should have been tested with the same or similar target population.

Logan et al. (2004)
The following outcomes (dependent variables) were measured:

- Activities of living. The researchers provide evidence that the Barthel index and Nottingham EADL scales are valid and reliable when applied to the target population (stroke patients).
- Psychological well-being. The 12-item General Health Questionnaire (GHQ) was confirmed as valid and reliable in the general population.
- Ability to get out of the house was based on two items.
  1. The answer to the question: 'Do you get out of the house as much as you would like?'
     Validity: Is this a measure of outings or desire?
     Reliability: Are responses subject to extraneous influences, such as family support or emotional change? Did recruitment from care homes impose structural constraints on people's ability to get out as much as they wanted?
     Sensitivity: 'Yes' or 'no' responses appear to be used, whereas a scaled response might have been more sensitive to change.
  2. Self-reported number of outdoor journeys in the last month.
     Reliability: Is memory likely to affect accuracy?
     Validity: Is the response likely to be inflated if the participant is satisfied with the outcome?

A measure tested with one target population may not be valid, reliable or sensitive when applied to another. For example, Harwood and Ebrahim (2002) showed that the EADL was reliable when used with stroke patients, but not those undergoing hip replacement.

It is a good idea to check the validity and reliability (psychometric properties) of the principal outcome measures. Common measures are reviewed in reference books (e.g. Bowling 2005). Others are usually available to view (if not download) on the internet so you can apply your professional judgement.

Review notes:
Is there evidence that the measures used are valid, reliable and sensitive to change when used with this particular target population?
Review the measures and consider the validity and reliability of the outcomes in the context of the study and its target population.

Planned data analysis

The method of data analysis should be determined at the planning stage and details given in the Method section. The choice of statistical test is determined by the number of groups to be compared (in the case of Logan et al., two groups) and the type and distribution of the outcome measures (see Chapters 11, 12 and 14).

Review note:
Make a note of the statistical tests planned – this will help you make sense of the results.

Results

The results of an RCT follow a typical pattern:

• descriptive statistics and comparison of baseline measures;
• use of inferential statistical tests to compare group outcomes.

It is sensible to approach the review step by step.

Step 1: Check the type and distribution of outcome measurements

Descriptive statistics enable the reviewer to do the following:

1. Compare the study sample with known characteristics of the target population.
2. Become familiar with the scale of measurement (type of data) for each variable (see Chapter 3): is it categorical, continuous or ordinal?
3. Ascertain the distribution of the data for each variable (see Chapters 4 and 5). In the case of continuous data (Chapter 4), do the data approximate to the normal distribution?
4. Judge the appropriateness of the statistics used to describe the data and compare demographic and baseline data, based on the type and distribution of the outcome (dependent) variables (see Table 1.2).

Logan et al. (2004)
Two types of data were collected:

• categorical data, mostly dichotomous (consisting of two mutually exclusive categories), e.g. sex (male/female), gets out of the house as much as wants (yes/no);
• continuous data, including age in years, months since stroke, and activities of living and quality of life measurements.[3]

---

3 Individual responses regarding quality of life and activities of living are usually measured using ordinal scales, but when summed these are usually treated as continuous measurements.

Table 1.2 Types of data and tests of comparison

	Categorical data	Ordinal data	Continuous data	
Definition	Count of the number of cases or observations in each mutually exclusive category	Scale based on sequential categories, not separated by equal intervals (e.g. verbal rating scales)	Normally has at least 11 equidistant scale points (e.g. 0–10)	
Distribution requirements	Minimum cell counts are required for statistical testing	Not critical	Does not conform to the normal distribution	Conforms to the normal distribution
Descriptive statistics	Numbers Percentages	Nonparametric: Range Median Percentiles		Parametric: Range Mean Standard deviations
Baseline comparisons: 2 groups	Fisher exact test; Chi-square	Mann–Whitney U test		t test
Baseline comparisons: 3+ groups	Chi-square	Kruskal–Wallis		One-way ANOVA

Categorical data are described using numbers and percentages.

Logan et al. (2004)
The table of baseline data show that 24/86 (28%) of respondents in the intervention group reported being able to get out of the house as much as they wanted, compared to 32/82 (39%) in the control group (see extract in Table 1.3). These data are more easily understood when translated into a bar chart (see Figure 1.2).

Table 1.3 Ability to get out at baseline (from Logan et al. 2004)

	Intervention group (n = 86)	Control group (n = 82)
Able to get out at baseline	24 (28)	32 (39)

n refers to the number of participants in each category.
Percentages are given in brackets.

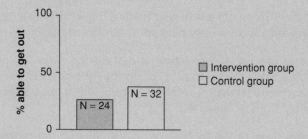

Figure 1.2 Bar chart of ability to get out (based on data from Logan et al. 2004)

Bar charts are easier to understand, but take up valuable space and are rarely used in an RCT report. You might find it helpful to construct your own (as we have done).

Continuous data (see Chapter 3) normally refer to a scale with at least 11 equidistant intervals (e.g. a 0–10 numerical scale). Continuous data that approximate to the normal distribution (see Chapter 4) are described and analysed using parametric statistics (those based on the normal distribution curve). Descriptive statistics include:

Range: indicated by the highest and lowest recorded values.

Mean: numerical average, calculated by summing up each value and dividing by the total number of observations (n).

Standard deviation: a standardised measure of variation of the data around the mean, given in the original units of measurement. Properties of the normal distribution curve predict that approximately 95% of the population will record a value of [mean ± 2 standard deviations].

Logan et al. (2004)

The mean age of the intervention group was 74 years, with a standard deviation of 8.4 years.

Assuming that the data conform to the normal distribution, we can calculate that approximately 95% of the sample will be aged:

Mean age ± 2 sd = 74 ± (2 × 8.4) = 57.2 to 90.8.

This means that less than 5% will be aged under 57 or over 91 years.

How can the reviewer tell if continuous data conform to
the normal distribution?

Before using parametric statistics, the researchers must ensure that the data approximate to the normal distribution. The following problems may arise:

Skewness: measurements are biased toward one end of the range.

Kurtosis: the data show a very peaked or flat distribution.

Researchers may use visual inspection and statistical tests for normality (see Chapter 4). Occasionally the assumption of normality is violated, which invalidates the use of parametric statistical tests. Therefore, it is a good idea to check the baseline data for signs of skewness:

1. The mean lies close to the highest or lowest value in the range, rather than close to the mid-point.

2. Add the standard deviation to the mean and subtract it from the mean (mean ± 1 sd). If either result lies outside the actual or possible range of recorded values, the data are extremely skewed.

3. Now calculate (mean ± 2 sd). If either result lies outside the actual or possible range of values, the data are somewhat skewed (as illustrated in Figure 1.3, where the value of −2 sd lies outside the possible range).

4. Where both values are given, skewness is indicated by a discrepancy between the mean and the median, as in Figure 1.3. (The median is the middle value when all values are placed in ascending order; see Chapter 4.) Statistical tests for skewness are based on this difference.

Logan et al. (2004)
'Mean time since stroke' at baseline in the control group is given as 10 months, with a standard deviation of 9 months.

The properties of the normal distribution predict that about 95% of the sample had their stroke between −8 months and +28 months ago (mean ± 2 sd). A value of −8 months is not possible, confirming that the data are somewhat skewed.

Our interpretation of the data, based on the values for control group mean (10 months) and standard deviation (9 months), plus our clinical experience, suggests a distribution similar to the illustration in Figure 1.3, on which the normal distribution curve is superimposed.

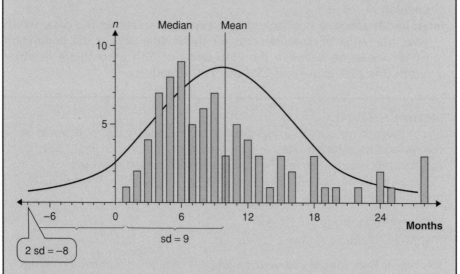

Figure 1.3 Interpretation of 'time since stroke' (based on control group data from Logan et al. 2004)

If the data do not approximate to the normal distribution, the researchers should apply nonparametric statistics (see Chapter 5).

Review notes:
Check that the researchers have reported on their inspections of the distribution of the data. If not, look carefully at the means and standard deviations of continuous data to see if any look 'skewed'.
Make a note to check that parametric statistical tests were not applied to variables that did not approximate to the normal distribution.

Nonparametric data are data that do not conform to the normal distribution including ordinal data (such as an individual verbal rating scale) and continuous data that fail to approximate to the normal distribution (see Table 1.2).

Instead of using numerical scores, nonparametric statistics are based on the rank position of each participant in the hierarchy of recorded values for each variable (see Chapter 5).

Nonparametric descriptive statistics include the following:

Range: highest and lowest recorded values for each variable.
Median: the middle value when individual scores are arranged in ascending order.
Percentiles: percentile represents the percentage of the sample or population with scores below the stated value.
Quartiles: the scores that mark the highest and lowest 25% of the sample or population.
Interquartile range: a nonparametric measure of spread in the data, which gives the range of measurements for the middle 50% of the population whose values lie between the 25th and the 75th percentile – in other words, the 25% above and 25% below the median.

Logan et al. (2004)
The number of outdoor journeys during the last month was reported to be skewed and therefore treated as nonparametric data. Accordingly, descriptive statistics give values for the median and interquartile range.

Logan et al. do not give baseline data for this variable, so our illustration uses data taken at 4-month follow-up:

• intervention group: 37 (18–62)

• control group: 14 (5–34)

This means that, for the intervention group, the median number of outings was 37, with 50% going out between 18 and 62 times. For the control group, the median number of outings was 14, with 50% going out between 5 and 34 times.

Review note:
Check that the descriptive statistics are compatible with the type and distribution of the data. Make a note of any discrepancies.

Step 2: Compare demographic and baseline measurements

The next task is to check that there were no statistically significant differences between the intervention and control groups at baseline on any demographic or baseline variables. A significant difference indicates that randomisation was not successful and the outcome potentially biased.

The researchers usually present baseline measurements in the form of a table of comparison. Guidance on the choice of statistical test for baseline comparisons was given in Table 1.2 (p. 15). To help you with your own review, our illustrations include each type of data.

Comparing categorical baseline data

Logan et al. (2004)

Table 1.4 Categorical baseline measurements (based on Logan et al. 2004)

Dependent variables	Intervention group n (%)	Control group n (%)
Men	40 (46%)	51 (62%)
Gets out of house as much as wants	24 (28%)	32 (39%)

The baseline measures in Table 1.4 do not appear identical but statistical tests of difference were not reported, as we should have expected. Using Table 1.2, the appropriate statistical test of comparison where there are two groups is either the Fisher exact test or the chi-square test.

We applied the simple formula for chi-square (χ^2) by hand (see Chapter 11 for details) and our results showed the following:

1. There was a significant difference between the number of men in each group ($\chi^2 = 5.13$, $p \leq 0.05$). This could bias the findings if there was reason to suppose that men might respond differently than women to the intervention or the person delivering it.
2. There was no statistical group difference in the number of people able to get out of the house as much as they wanted ($\chi^2 = 2.33$, $p > 0.05$).[4]

Where statistical differences in demographic or baseline measures exist, the researchers should use statistical procedures to control for them in subsequent analyses, or take account of them in drawing a conclusion about the results.

---

4 A *p* value greater than 0.05 (*p* > 0.05) is not statistically significant.

Comparing continuous baseline data

Where continuous demographic or baseline measures have a normal distribution, it is usual to present these as a table of means and standard deviations, as in Table 1.5.

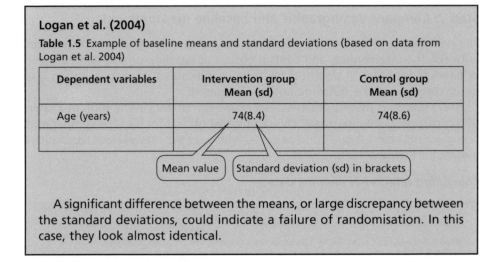

Logan et al. (2004)

Table 1.5 Example of baseline means and standard deviations (based on data from Logan et al. 2004)

Dependent variables	Intervention group Mean (sd)	Control group Mean (sd)
Age (years)	74(8.4)	74(8.6)

Mean value   Standard deviation (sd) in brackets

A significant difference between the means, or large discrepancy between the standard deviations, could indicate a failure of randomisation. In this case, they look almost identical.

If a difference between group means is suspected, but not confirmed, it is easy to test this using the formula for the unrelated *t* test (see Chapter 11):

$$t = \frac{\text{mean (group 1)} - \text{mean (group 2)}}{\text{pooled standard deviation}}.$$

The resulting value of *t* is checked against the statistical table of critical values of *t*,[5] as in Table 1.6, to ascertain statistical significance.

Table 1.6 Extract from a table of 'critical values' of *t*

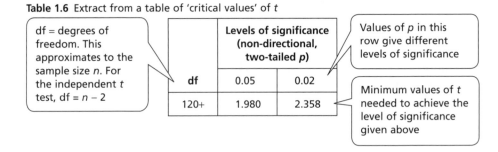

df = degrees of freedom. This approximates to the sample size *n*. For the independent *t* test, df = *n* − 2

	Levels of significance (non-directional, two-tailed *p*)	
df	0.05	0.02
120+	1.980	2.358

Values of *p* in this row give different levels of significance

Minimum values of *t* needed to achieve the level of significance given above

---

5   A critical value is the minimum value of the test statistic to achieve significance at the level of probability indicated. Statistical tables used to be the only method of interpreting statistical results before the advent of computerised statistical packages. They are found at the back of most basic textbooks on statistics. A useful web-based source is http://www.statsoft.com/textbook/sttable.htm.

If $n > 120$ and the significance level is set at $p \leq 0.05$, a value of $t \geq 1.98$ is required to demonstrate a statistically significant baseline difference in age between the intervention and the control group.

Nonparametric baseline comparisons

If the data are ordinal, or continuous but fail to conform to the normal distribution (see Chapter 4), the Mann–Whitney U test replaces the t test as the appropriate test of group difference (see Table 1.2).

Logan et al. (2004)
Baseline scores for the GHQ and activities of living are given as median and interquartile range (see Table 1.7), presumably because the data were skewed (though the researchers give no direct evidence to support this).

Table 1.7 Example of a table containing median and interquartile range (based on data from Logan et al. 2004)

Dependent variables	Intervention group Median (interquartile range)	Control group Median (interquartile range)
Barthel index	18 (16–20)	17 (13–20)
Nottingham EADL	23 (12–30)	21 (9–35)
GHQ	10 (7–13)	11 (8–13)

The median is the middle value when all measurements are placed in ascending order.

The interquartile range refers to the values that encompass the 25% of people who scored above the median and the 25% below the median.

The Mann–Whitney U test is based on raw data which are not available to the reviewer to check. The only option is to look carefully at the data to see if the median and range values are reasonably comparable.

Review notes:
Look at the baseline data to ensure that the type and distribution of the data are compatible with the descriptive statistics used. For example, if means and standard deviations were used, do the data appear to approximate to the normal distribution?
Are there any obvious discrepancies between the groups? Did the researchers test for statistically significant differences between the intervention and control groups at baseline? Where possible, if you are not satisfied, do your own check to see if any differences are statistically different. What might be the reason for any discrepancy?

Step 3: Comparing group outcomes

The final task is to check that appropriate tests were used to identify any statistical differences in outcome between the intervention group and the control group. The key checks are as follows:

1. The statistical tests must address the original research questions or hypotheses.
2. The selected statistical tests of group difference must be compatible with the type and distribution of the data (see Step 2 on baseline data).

Logan et al. (2004)
The primary objective was to improve mobility using four types of measurement:

1. The ability to get out of the house as much as they wanted: yes or no. This is a dichotomous variable.
2. Number of outdoor journeys undertaken during the last month. This was a continuous measure, but the data were skewed.
3. Self-report of mobility. This measure contains three discrete categories of response: housebound, travels accompanied, travels unaccompanied.
4. Nottingham EADL mobility subscale, measured using a continuous scale.

The secondary objective was to establish if the intervention improved quality of life, measured using three continuous measures:

1. the Barthel index;
2. the Nottingham EADL scale, total plus three additional subscales of unknown distributions (kitchen, domestic, leisure);
3. the GHQ, which appears to have a normal distribution.

Statistical tests used to compare outcomes are usually more complex than those used to compare baseline measures because they need to answer two questions, preferably at the same time:

- Did the measures for the intervention group show significant improvement from baseline to follow-up?
- Assuming measurements were the same at baseline, were the outcomes at follow-up significantly better in the intervention group than the control group?

The most common methods of analysis used in RCTs are as follows:

- Test the effect of the intervention using predetermined criteria to classify the outcome as either successful or unsuccessful (a dichotomous outcome measure). For example, ability to get out of the house.
- Test for changes and differences using a continuous outcome scale, such as those used to measure quality of life.

Comparing ability to get out of the house
This measure is categorical and is termed dichotomous because it consists of a single characteristic that is either present or absent (see Table 1.8).

Logan et al. (2004)

Table 1.8 Example of a table of categorical data (from Logan et al. 2004)

	Able to get out at baseline	Able to get out by 4 months	Able to get out by 10 months
Intervention group, n = 86 (%)	24 (28%)	56 (65%)	53 (62%)
Control group, n = 82 (%)	32 (39%)	30 (35%)	33 (38%)

We constructed a graph of these data to make the outcome easier to envisage. We encourage you to do likewise when reviewing these types of data (see Figure 1.4). While the control group remained relatively unchanged over time, there is a marked increase in the ability of the intervention group to get out by 4 months, maintained at 10 months.

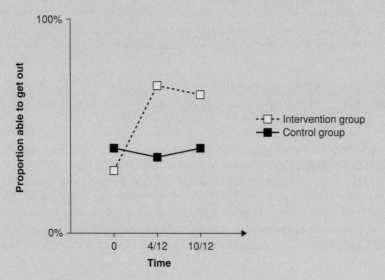

Figure 1.4 Graph of proportions able to get out at baseline and follow-up (based on data from Logan et al. 2004)

Two tests of statistical significance may be used to compare the two groups using a dichotomous variable: the Fisher exact test or chi-square. In fact, a more effective method for presenting this type of result is using relative risk (RR) followed, if statistically significant, by number needed to treat (NNT) (see Chapter 16), as shown in Table 1.9.

Logan et al. (2004)

Table 1.9 Table of results giving relative risk and number needed to treat
(from Logan et al. 2004)

	Able to get out (intervention group, $n = 86$)	Able to get out (control group, $n = 82$)	Relative risk (95% CI)	Number needed to treat (NNT)
4 month follow-up	56	30	1.72 (1.25 to 2.37)	3.3
10 month follow-up	53	33	1.74 (1.24 to 2.44)	4.0

Statistical significance is indicated if both values for the confidence interval (CI) are greater than 1

Number of patients who need to be treated in order to achieve one successful outcome

We note that according to errata and corrections given in the following issue of the *British Medical Journal*, these figures were reported incorrectly. However, we have used data from the original article here.

In this context, relative risk refers to the proportion of the intervention group that benefited, compared to the proportion in the control group that benefited. Using the example of data from the 10-month follow-up, the calculation is:

Proportion of the intervention group able to get out = 53/86 = 0.6163.

Proportion of the control group able to get out = 33/82 = 0.4024.

Relative risk (benefit) = 0.6163 ÷ 0.4024 = 1.53.[6]

Assuming the significance level is set at $\alpha = 0.05$ (i.e. $p \leq 0.05$), a statistically significant difference between groups is indicated if both values for the 95% confidence interval (CI) for RR are either greater than 1 or less than –1.[7]

Number needed to treat (NNT) is only relevant if the relative benefit of the intervention is statistically significant. NNT is calculated as $1/x$ where x is the difference between the proportions of each group who benefited:

---

6 We note a discrepancy between our calculation of RR (1.53) and the figure given by Logan et al. (1.74). Errata and corrections to this research paper were published in the next edition of the *British Medical Journal*, though these did not entirely address our concerns regarding this discrepancy.

7 The 95% CI gives the range of values within which the true value will be found 95% of the time. Our significance level is 95%; the significance level and α are complementary such that the significance level equals $1 - \alpha$; here $\alpha = 1 - 0.05 = 0.05$. CI is given as a percentage; alpha or p is given in decimals.

Proportion of the intervention group able to get out = 53/86 = 0.6163

Proportion of the control group able to get out = 33/82 = 0.4024

Difference in proportions able to get out (NNT) = $1 \div (0.62 \times 0.40) = 4.03$.

Logan et al. report the NNT as 4, which implies that at least 4 people would need to receive the OT intervention in order for one person to benefit in terms of getting out.

The closer the value of NNT to 1, the more effective the treatment. Importantly, we should have expected Logan et al. to give a 95% CI for the value for NNT, since NNT is an estimate and not a precise figure.

Relative risk versus odds ratio

Some researchers prefer to give the odds ratio (OR) instead of the relative risk (see Chapter 16). The odds ratio refers to the ratio of the odds of an event occurring in one group, compared to the odds of it occurring in another group.

Logan et al. (2004)

The odds ratio is calculated thus:

- In the intervention group, the ratio of those able to get out, compared to those not able to get out at 10 months, is $53 \div 33 = 1.6$.
- In the control group, the ratio is $33 \div 49 = 0.67$.
- Odds ratio (OR) = $1.6 \div 0.67 = 2.4$.

As with relative risk, if both values for the 95% CI are greater than 1 (or less than −1), the difference in outcome between groups is statistically significant ($p \leq 0.05$).

OR is interpreted in the same way as RR, though it tends to inflate the outcome when compared to RR.

Review notes:

If the researchers have given details of relative risk or odds ratio and number needed to treat, have they included the appropriate confidence interval for each measure?

Look at the lower limit of the CI – is the result statistically significant (i.e. greater than 1 or less than −1)? Are you impressed with these results? Would you recommend that your own unit invest in an intervention likely to yield results of this magnitude?

Does the number needed to treat suggest that the intervention might prove cost-effective?

Comparing improvements in quality of life, based on GHQ scores
A large number of RCTs use outcome measures, such as the GHQ, that are continuous and known to conform to the normal distribution in the general population. Group differences are usually analysed using analysis of variance (ANOVA) to answer the question: is there a statistically significant improvement in outcome between baseline and follow-up in the intervention group, when compared to the control group?

In the Logan et al. study, the use of baseline medians and interquartile range indicates that their data did not conform to the normal distribution. However, we have introduced additional assumptions to illustrate the use of ANOVA using their data.

Analysis of variance
ANOVA (see Chapter 12) is a parametric test that measures between-group differences at follow-up while taking account of within-group improvements between baseline and follow-up.

Key assumptions of ANOVA (see Chapter 14) include the following:

- The outcome measure is continuous and the data conform to the normal distribution.
- Standard deviations for each group are roughly the same.

Logan et al. (2004)
We have substituted means and standard deviations for the medians and interquartile ranges given by Logan et al., and assumed that the data approximate to the normal distribution (see Table 1.10). A graph helps visualise these data. It is worth constructing one, as in Figure 1.5, if the researchers have not done so.

Table 1.10 Table of means and standard deviations

GHQ scores	Intervention group ($n = 86$) Mean (sd)	Control group ($n = 82$) Mean (sd)
Baseline	10 (3.5)	11 (3.5)
4 months	16 (4.0)	12 (3.7)
10 months	14 (3.9)	11.5 (3.6)

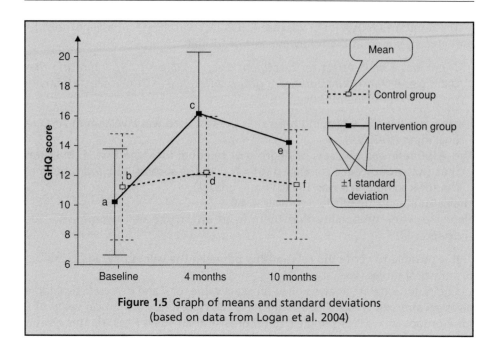

Figure 1.5 Graph of means and standard deviations
(based on data from Logan et al. 2004)

Figure 1.5 illustrates the mean difference and the extent of overlap between GHQ scores for each group at each point in time. It shows that the groups started out with very similar baseline measurements, but while scores for the control group stayed much the same over time, scores for the intervention group increased and then reduced slightly.

If there are any demographic or baseline differences following randomisation, it is possible to control for these by including them as covariates in a version of ANOVA called analysis of covariance (ANCOVA). A research question answered using ANCOVA might be: 'allowing for differences in baseline mobility, did the intervention lead to a statistically significant improvement in GHQ scores at follow-up when compared to the control group?'

ANOVA and ANCOVA give the following results:

- **Main effect for groups.** Between-group differences are represented in Figure 1.5 by differences between the mean scores for the intervention and control groups at each point in time: *a* versus *b*, *c* versus *d*, and *e* versus *f*.

- **Main effects for time.** Within-group changes are represented in Figure 1.5 by differences between the following means: for the control group, *b* versus *d*, *d* versus *f*, and *b* versus *f*; and for the intervention group, *a* versus *c*, *c* versus *e*, and *a* versus *e*.

Interaction between intervention and time is illustrated by the extent of any cross-over or divergence of the connecting lines on the graph.

The results of ANOVA (or in this case ANCOVA, controlling for baseline mobility) are typically stated in the following sort of format:

There was a main effect for treatment ($F_{1,166} = 4.0$, $p \leq 0.05$), indicating that there was a statistically significant group difference in GHQ scores, after controlling for baseline mobility.

F is the test statistic, which indicates that the test used was a version of ANOVA (including ANCOVA).

The 1,166 refers to two sets of degrees of freedom (df):[8] the first, 1, indicates that two groups were compared (df = n – 1); the second, 166, indicates that the total sample size was 168 (df = n – groups).

The calculated value of the F statistic is 4.0.

Finally, p is the probability that there is *no* effect (the null hypothesis – see Chapter 9).

It is possible to verify the relationship between the values of F and p in a set of statistical tables (see Table 1.11).

Computerised data analysis gives an exact value for F and p. A statistical table gives an approximation. From Table 1.11, the closest (lower) critical value of F for 2 groups (df = 1) for sample size (n) greater than 150 is $F \geq 3.91$. This gives $p = 0.05$, which is statistically significant. [Note that tables for F values assume a two-tailed test of probability.] This confirms that $F_{1,166} = 4.0$ is statistically significant ($p \leq 0.05$).

Table 1.11 Extract from statistical table for F

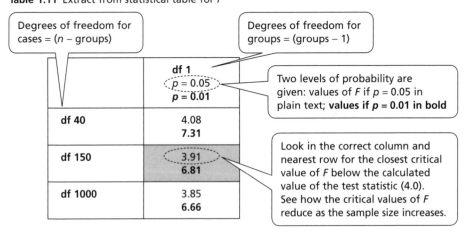

---

8 Degrees of freedom are closely related to the size of the data set, but contain statistical adjustments to reduce overestimating statistical significance.

Post-hoc multiple comparisons
ANOVA does not specify exactly where the main effects are. Does the difference between groups occur at 4 months (c versus d in Figure 1.5) or at 10 months (e versus f) or both?

Once a statistically significant main effect is established using ANOVA, multiple 'post hoc' tests of comparison identify the precise sources of difference (see chapter 14 for more details of these tests).

Frequently Asked Questions (FAQs)

1. *Why should researchers bother with ANOVA? Why not just use multiple t tests to analyse differences between groups at follow-up, and within-group changes?*
Some researchers do this, but it is actually cheating since the results are susceptible to false positive findings (Type I error). Multiple tests of comparison should be conducted only after achieving a significant result using ANOVA.

2. *What is the nonparametric equivalent of ANOVA for clinical trial data that do not approximate to the normal distribution?*
There isn't one. Friedman two-way ANOVA by ranks is actually only capable of comparing repeated measurements within a single group. If the data are nonparametric, it is necessary to include multiple tests of group comparison, but the significance level should be reduced from $\alpha = 0.05$ to, say, $\alpha = 0.01$ (e.g. using the Bonferroni correction – see Chapter 9) to reduce the likelihood of Type I error.

3. *Are there any equivalent methods of analysis that can be used for categorical and nonparametric data?*
There is no alternative test of group difference. However, logistic regression is a form of multidimensional contingency table used to identify the combination of continuous and categorical variables that distinguish between a successful and unsuccessful outcome. Logan et al. used this method to identify variables that predicted a difference between the intervention group and the control group.[9]

We illustrate nonparametric analyses in the following sections.

---

9 In their section on statistical analysis, Logan et al. say they used 'linear multiple regression'. But multiple regression requires a continuous, normally distributed outcome measure. The outcome measure specified (self-reported mobility) consists of three categories, therefore we assume that they actually mean to say logistic regression (though we are not clear that the sample size was powered for this purpose).

Review notes:
Do the researchers give means and standard deviations for all baseline and follow-up data measured using a continuous scale?
Were all of the assumptions of ANOVA fulfilled, notably those relating to the normal distribution and homogeneity of variance?
Were multiple group comparisons carried out after ANOVA confirmed statistical significance?

Comparing the number of outdoor journeys made during the last month

Logan et al. (2004)
This outcome measure is continuous but the data are skewed (see Table 1.12). Median values for each group suggest differences between the intervention and control groups at 4 and at 10 months, while the control group means remained unchanged during this period.

Table 1.12 Results for number of outdoor journeys (based on Logan et al. 2004)

Outdoor journeys in past month	Intervention group Median (interquartile range)	Control group Median (interquartile range)
4 months	37 (18–62)	14 (5–34)
10 months	42 (13–69)	14 (7–32)

However, the interquartile range values indicate greater variation in values for the intervention group (13–69 at 10 months) than for the control group (7–32). Also, the distribution of values is skewed in the control group but not in the intervention group (in a normal distribution the median would be at the mid-point of the interquartile range). This makes it difficult for the reviewer to make a direct comparison or judge if the difference is statistically significant.

Logan et al. correctly used nonparametric statistics to compare the groups at follow-up using the Mann–Whitney U test (see Table 1.2 and also Chapter 11). The results at 4 and 10 months are given as $p < 0.01$, which indicates a chance of less than a 1 in 100 that there is *no* difference between the number of outdoor journeys taken by the members of the two groups (statistical tests always test the null hypothesis). This confirms a statistically significant difference between groups at each follow-up point.

Should we be impressed by this result? After all, the Mann–Whitney U test only compares group outcomes at a single point in time and does not take account of relative change over time. We looked for other clues in the data:

- The lack of baseline data for this variable makes it difficult to ascertain overall improvement. However, the consistency of medians and interquartile variations for the number of outings in the control group over the study period suggest that the control group data probably reflect a reasonable estimate of baseline values.
- It seems unlikely that the intervention group started out with any advantage since, as a group, they were less satisfied with the number of outings at baseline.
- The results for both perceived and actual outings in the intervention group were sustained between 4-month and 10-month follow-up.

These observations all confirm enduring benefit from the intervention.

Review notes:
When evaluating the results, don't just look at the value of p. Look carefully at the values given, such as percentages, median and interquartile range, or means and standard deviations, at different points in the study. Look critically at the information given and the meaning of the data:

- *Do the researchers give complete data for baseline and follow-ups?*
- *What does the pattern of results appear to indicate about the effect and sustainability of the outcome?*

Comparing secondary outcomes: activities of living and quality of life

The secondary outcome of the Logan et al. study was to assess impact on activities of living and quality of life using the Nottingham EADL scales (mobility, kitchen use, domestic activity and leisure), and scores on the GHQ. The researchers wanted to control for factors that might have biased the outcomes:

'We used multivariate linear regression analysis to analyse the secondary outcome measures. This analysis was adjusted for baseline variables (sex, ethnic origin, age, prior use of transport).' (p. 1373)

Their use of the term 'multivariate linear regression' is confusing since it fails to distinguish between multiple regression and logistic regression.

Multiple regression is a parametric test, similar to ANCOVA in many respects. We can be sure that Logan et al. did not use this test because the results are not given. Further, the results are not given in the format for multiple regression (see Chapter 16 and the worked example in Chapter 2).

We assume that the test used was logistic regression. This is a nonparametric test used to determine the ability of a range of independent variables, regardless of type and distribution, to predict the occurrence or non-occurrence of an event – in this case improvement versus no improvement.

The term 'covariate' signals the use of statistical control, as in ANCOVA. The covariates are variables introduced first into the regression equation to eliminate their potentially biasing effect on outcomes.

In Figure 1.6 we focus on results for the EADL total score and the mobility subscale score. Logan et al. present the results in the form of a 'forest plot', which is increasingly popular and relatively easy to understand.

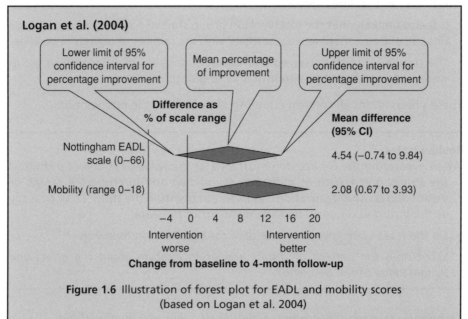

Figure 1.6 Illustration of forest plot for EADL and mobility scores (based on Logan et al. 2004)

In a forest plot, the mean difference between groups is indicated by the fat midpoint of the diamond, and the confidence interval by the horizontal endpoints.[10]

- If both values for the confidence interval are on the same side of 0, there is a statistically significant difference between groups such that the improvement in one group outweighs those in the other group (check the direction to see which group is favoured).
- If any part of the diamond straddles 0, the difference between groups is not statistically significant.

The (correct) results show that the intervention demonstrated a significant improvement in EADL mobility subscale scores over standard care, but there was no statistically significant improvement using the EADL total score.

We note that, in this paper, GHQ scores for carers were introduced into the results even though this was never mentioned in the aim, introduction or hypotheses.

---

10 Note that the values on the horizontal axis are not consistent with the confidence intervals – errata were subsequently printed in a later issue of the *British Medical Journal*.

Review notes:
Were the researchers clear about the method of statistical analysis used?
Did they explain and justify the methods used?
Were the results presented in a way that was comprehensible?
Did the statistical tests focus only on hypotheses developed in the Introduction?

Discussion and conclusions

The final task is to ensure that the researchers give an accurate account of the results and have taken into account any potential biases when presenting their conclusions.

Logan et al. (2004)
Logan et al. focus their discussion on the sustained improvements in mobility as a result of the intervention. They note that this is based on self-report measures which, though susceptible to bias, have the advantage of being personally relevant.
 There were no secondary effects in terms of improvement in quality of life. One possible reason given is the small sample size, though this is really no excuse as the original sample size calculation should have made adequate allowance for this analysis.

Review notes:
Do the researchers consider all of the potential biases that you have noted in your review?
Do they focus only on the original hypotheses and results or do they introduce new issues into their discussion and conclusions?
Do the researchers base their conclusions only on results that were statistically significant?
Are acceptable reasons given for the failure to find support for hypotheses?
Is the use of language used to convey the conclusions compatible with the strength of the statistical results?

Conclusions from our survey review

If you have recorded review notes, compare your appraisal of the Logan et al. survey with our ideas below.

Logan et al. (2004)

Overall, this is an interesting study that focused on an important issue for public health practice, notably that of improving mobility and quality of life following stroke.

The primary outcome demonstrated significant gains of considerable magnitude in the intervention group, compared to the control group, using self-reported measures of mobility. However, the study may have been compromised by including patients of varying ages and post-stroke durations; the study failed to control for additional professional attention; the study was underpowered and the sample size possibly too small to detect statistically significant results on all measures; some principal outcome measures had not been subject to adequate checks for validity, reliability or clinical relevance.

The report of regression analysis is confusing and a number of other errors in the results were reported after publication. The 95% confidence interval for number needed to treat is an important omission.

Nevertheless the results suggest a sustained improvement in mobility following the intervention compared to a total absence of improvement on any measure among stroke patients receiving usual care.

Further study, including cost–benefit analysis, would be required before it was worth investing in this intervention.

2 The Health Survey

Introduction

Health surveys are widely used to collect and analyse health-related information. The findings enhance our understanding of a wide range of factors that contribute to health and well-being among different population groups in various settings. This chapter is based on the following example which you will find in boxes throughout the chapter as illustrated below.

> **Chisholm et al. (2007)**
> Chisholm, V., Atkinson, L., Donaldson, C., Noyes, K., Payne, A. and Kelnar, C. (2007) Predictors of treatment adherence in young children with type 1 diabetes. *Journal of Advanced Nursing*, 57(5): 482–493.

Types of health survey

There are three main types of survey used in health care research.

Epidemiological surveys are typically used to:

- describe health status (e.g. the prevalence of a disease or set of symptoms or disability in different population groups);
- determine demographic and lifestyle discriminators for health and disease (e.g. age, gender, smoking, treatment adherence).

Epidemiological surveys commonly combine objective medical data with self-report data to enhance validity.

Social surveys are typically used to:

- describe public knowledge, beliefs and attitudes about important health issues;
- develop theoretical associations between these factors and health status and/or quality of life.

Social surveys are based on self-report data and focus on abstract concepts such as 'well-being' and 'quality of life' that require valid and reliable methods of measurement (see Chapter 6).

Satisfaction surveys are typically used to:

- describe public attitudes and opinions towards health and/or health and social care.

These are similar to market surveys, but are often small scale and rarely based on a random sample.

Each type of survey may be primarily descriptive (use descriptive statistics to characterise the target population) or analytic (use inferential statistics to identify predictors of health status in the target population) or both.

> **Chisholm et al. (2007)**
> Chisholm et al. (2007) combined epidemiological with social survey methods. Their primary aim was analytic: to identify predictors of adherence. Accordingly, they use inferential statistics to identify predictors of treatment adherence in young children with type 1 diabetes.

Review note:
Identify the type of survey used.
Is the purpose descriptive or analytic or both?

The research aim, questions and hypotheses

The purpose of the study should be stated at the beginning of the introduction to orientate the reader. Specific research questions, objectives or hypotheses emerge from an appraisal of the literature and are usually found at the end of the introduction or literature review.

- An **aim** is a broad statement of intention.
- A **research question** is an explicit or implicit question that the research is designed to address.
- An **objective** is a statement of intention about a course of action to be achieved as part of the research.
- A **hypothesis** is an explicit or implicit prediction of the likely finding or outcome, based on clearly defined theory or existing research-based evidence.

The research questions, objectives and hypotheses determine the statistical tests used to analyse the data (see Chapter 9 on hypothesis testing). They also influence the test of probability applied to the statistical test results.

> **Chisholm et al. (2007)**
> The aim of the Chisholm et al. study is encapsulated within the title, stated in the abstract and restated at the start of the Method section, in a subsection entitled 'The study' (p. 484):
>
> *'The aim of the study was to investigate whether diabetes-specific, demographic and psychosocial variables predicted adherence in young children with T1D [Type 1 diabetes]'*
>
> A blanket hypothesis is implicit within the research aim: there *may be* an association between diabetes-specific, demographic and psychosocial variables and variables that measure adherence.

Note that the researchers predict there *may be* an association. This use of language determines the test of probability applied to the statistical results (see Chapter 9):

- A confident (directional) prediction about a relationship or outcome is tested using a directional or one-tailed test of probability. This is more likely to give a significant result and must be supported by sound theoretical or research-based evidence.
- A question or uncertain prediction is tested using a non-directional or two-tailed test of probability. This is less susceptible to a false significant result (Type II error).

Review notes:

Make a note of each research question and hypothesis identified in the Introduction. You will need to refer back to these when appraising the results and conclusions.

Consider the language used in the aim, research question, or hypothesis. Check the introductory section to see if directional predictions are clearly justified.

Make a note of the test of probability you expect to be applied to each research question or hypothesis.

The introduction, background or literature review

From a statistical perspective, this section serves the following purposes:

- to provide theoretical justification for the concepts to be measured as variables for data collection and analysis;
- to establish potential causal links between a set of predictor (independent) variables and outcome (dependent) variables;
- to identify theoretical and/or research-based evidence to support a one-tailed or two-tailed test of probability to test the relationship between the predictor and outcome variables.

Chisholm et al. (2007)
In their Introduction, Chisholm et al. consider the following:

Predictor variables

- Diabetes-specific knowledge
- Demographic variables including social class, sex, age and illness duration
- Psychosocial variables including psychological functioning, parenting stress and family environment

Outcome variables

- Adherence to injection-giving regime
- Adherence to blood glucose monitoring (BGM) regime
- Adherence to dietary regime.

Review notes:
Make a list of the predictor and dependent variables.
It is also a good idea to draw conceptual maps of the predicted relationships between these, as in Figure 2.1.
Record any discrepancies between the research questions or hypotheses and evidence in the literature.
Confirm the test of probability you expect to see applied to statistical tests in the Results section.

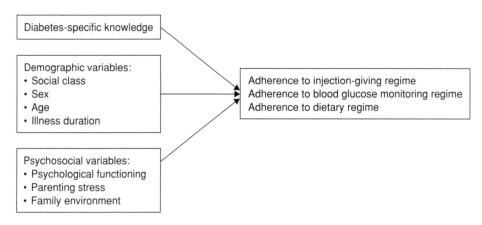

Figure 2.1 Predicted causal relationships between predictor and dependent variables

Chisholm et al. (2007)
Chisholm et al. review a range of potential predictors, but evidence for associations between these and adherence in children with type 1 diabetes is sparse. Therefore, a non-directional (two-tailed) test of probability should be applied to the statistical test results.

Research design

Surveys may be divided into three temporal types:

- **Cross-sectional surveys** provide a snapshot of what is happening now, as in the Chisholm et al. study.
- **Retrospective surveys** seek to identify what occurred at a specified time in the past.
- **Prospective surveys** involve taking repeated measurements from the same cohort over a period of time and requires 'repeated measures' statistical tests.

Data collection tools and methods

Data collection tools used in surveys include:

- questionnaires;
- structured interviews;
- documentary data;
- direct observation.

Questionnaires

Self-completion questionnaires are easy to administer, but rates of return in postal surveys can be as low as 12% (for possible reasons, see Chapter 8 on attrition).

Chisholm et al. (2007)
The following questionnaires were used:

- Diabetes Knowledge Questionnaire (DKQ), 53 items;
- Parenting Stress Index (PSI-SF), has 36 items;
- Family Environment Scale, number of items not easily obtainable;
- Child Behaviour Checklist (CBCL-P). Our internet search using Google indicated that the version for children aged 6–18 has 118 items (Achenbach 2008). Chisholm et al. do not state if all of these were used.

The burden imposed on mothers in this study was high. This could reduce the completeness of the data set, unless completion was supervised.

Structured interview

A structured interview schedule often includes the same measurement scales as a questionnaire, but has the advantage of a captive audience. The response rate may be high, but the approach can lead to social response bias.

Chisholm et al. (2007)
Telephone interviews were conducted with mothers to measure adherence, based on a 24-hour recall technique. We wonder if mothers would be reluctant to admit doing 'the wrong thing'. Therefore, we recommend examining whether the originators of this procedure (Johnson et al. 1986) checked for social response bias.

Documentary data

Documentary data include medical test results and other information taken from medical records. This is considered 'objective', provided it is accurately recorded and up to date.

> **Chisholm et al. (2007)**
> Medical records were used to collect demographic data, as well as objective data on duration of type 1 diabetes and measures of glycaemic control.

Direct observation

People tend to change their behaviour if they know they are being observed (Hawthorne effect). Therefore observation methods may require covert watching or video-recording (which introduce ethical challenges).

> **Chisholm et al. (2007)**
> The validity and reliability of adherence measures might have been strengthened had mothers been asked to record behaviours as they occurred, rather than relying on recall.

Review notes:
Were the methods of data collection the most appropriate ones that might have been selected?
Check for any conditions that might reduce the response rate or bias the findings.

Validity and reliability

No statistical test can compensate for measurement error, hence the need for rigorous checks on the validity and reliability of measures used (see Chapter 6).

> **Chisholm et al. (2007)**
> The measures of psychological functioning were reported to be 'internationally recognised self-report measures'.
>
> - Coefficient alpha scores (see Chapter 6 for explanation and criteria) for the PSI-SF and CBCL-P were reported to be greater than 0.85, indicating good internal consistency.
> - According to Chisholm et al., scores for the Family Environment Scale subscales range from $\alpha = 0.61$ (only just acceptable) to 0.78 (fairly good), with reliability 0.68 (acceptable) to 0.86 (good).
>
> We conducted our own investigation of the DKQ and found it difficult to locate details of its psychometric properties (validity and reliability). Chisholm et al. state that they constructed it from previous questionnaires designed originally for use with diabetic adults and included additional items related to younger children's care. This raises some doubts about its validity and reliability.

A reliable measure gives consistent results when used again in similar conditions.

> **Chisholm et al. (2007)**
> The child's HbA1c test result was used as a reliable measure of glycaemic control. A quick internet check using the search terms 'HbA1c', 'reliable' and 'diabetes' revealed recent evidence by Nishimura et al. (2008) that cast doubt on the validity and reliability of HbA1c as a measure of glycaemic control in adults. We were unable to find evidence concerning its use with children and would want to extend our search before drawing conclusions about its use in this context.

Review notes:
Does the researcher give adequate information about validity and reliability? Is it worth checking up on the measures used?
Has the measure been used previously with the same target population? If not, is it really applicable in the present research situation?

Sampling procedure

Survey methods involve one of the following types of sampling (described in detail in Chapter 7):

- **Population sample**: all those who meet the inclusion and exclusion criteria (the target population), e.g. all children in the UK with type 1 diabetes.
- **Random or probability sample**: a representative sample drawn at random from the target population.
- **Stratified random sample:** a separate random sample taken from each of two or more unequal size subgroups to facilitate statistical comparisons.
- **Cluster sample:** samples taken from different locations to ensure diverse representation within the target population, e.g. all children with type 1 diabetes attending selected GP practices representing diverse sites throughout the country (rural, urban, different levels of socio-economic status, etc.).
- **Purposive sampling:** used in qualitative research, this has no place in quantitative methods.
- **Convenience or opportunity sampling**: a haphazard process based on easily accessible members of the target population, often in a single location, e.g. children with type 1 diabetes attending a local clinic. The disadvantage is that the findings do not necessarily generalise to the target population.

> **Chisholm et al. (2007)**
> Chisholm et al. state that they recruited a convenience sample of children aged 2–8 attending a Scottish diabetes clinic.

Review notes:
What method of sampling was used?
If a large random sample was not used, look carefully at the demographic
characteristics and baseline data for clues that might differentiate the study
sample from known characteristics of the target population.
If convenience sampling was used, make a note to look carefully at the descriptive
statistics to see how representative the sample appears to be.

Sample size

Table 2.1 Recommended sample sizes for descriptive surveys

The dependent variable has at least an 11-point scale (e.g. 0–10) with equidistant intervals

Significance level/ size of confidence interval

The dependent variable consists of 2 or more mutually exclusive categories

Size of population to be represented	Sample size required ($\alpha = 0.05/95\%\,CI$)	
	Continuous data	Categorical data
100	55	80
500	96	218
1000	106	278
4000+	120	400

Figures are based on Bartlett et al. (2001).

Descriptive surveys

The sample size for a purely descriptive survey is based on the size of the target population (see Table 2.1).

> **Chisholm et al. (2007)**
> Had Chisholm et al. wished to ensure that descriptive characteristics from their sample would generalise to the population of children with type 1 diabetes in the UK, they would have needed a random sample of at least 120 children from across the UK, given that most of their independent and dependent variables were measured using a continuous scale.

Analytic surveys

The sample size for a survey that involves the use of inferential statistics needs to be calculated in advance to ensure a statistically significant result will be achieved, if there is one to be found. Table 2.2 suggests approximate *minimum* sample size recommendations, based on reasonable consensus from a number of sources.

Table 2.2 Rough guide to minimum sample sizes

Purpose	Continuous data	Categorical data[a]
Compare groups	$n \geq 15$ in each group	$n > 50$ (2 groups, 2 categories) $n > 60$ (2 groups, 3 categories)
Correlate 2 variables	$n \geq 30$	
Multivariate analysis	Multiple regression: $n \geq 100$ if there are up to 5 independent (predictor) variables Add 20 for each additional predictor	Logistic regression $n > 400$

[a] These numbers are based on the assumption that the data are likely to be reasonably evenly distributed across categories.

When looking at the results, It is important to look carefully at the number of complete sets of responses (n) for each analysis: n must be large enough to detect a statistically significant difference between groups or relationship between variables, if there is one to be found. Note that the value of n may vary throughout the Results section if individuals failed to answer one or more questions included in the analysis.

Statisticians can estimate the sample size requirement (see Chapter 8) based on the following factors:

- The type and distribution of the data collected, particularly the dependent variables.
  Parametric data are measured using a continuous (interval) numerical scale and conform to the pattern of the normal distribution (see Chapter 4). They are analysed using parametric statistics (based on the normal distribution curve).
  Nonparametric data are either continuous data that do not approximate to the normal distribution, or ordinal data, often those measured using a verbal rating scale, converted to a sequential numerical scale that does not assume equal intervals. Nonparametric statistics are based on the rank position of values in the data set, rather than the actual values (see Chapter 5).
  Categorical data consist of frequency counts recorded in mutually exclusive categories or cells in a 'contingency table' (see Chapter 11). Contingency analysis has minimum cell size requirements which necessitate larger sample sizes.
- The size of important subgroups to be compared. If the analysis involves comparing small population subgroups, such as an ethnic minority, the minimum sample size needs to be calculated for each group. For example, had Chisholm et al. compared adherence between different age groups, they might have ended up with a very small number at the lower end of the age spectrum. If these sorts of comparisons are planned, stratified sampling should be used to ensure adequate subgroup sizes.
- The type of statistical analysis planned. Multivariate analyses (those that analyse the combined effect of several predictor variables) require much larger sample sizes than simple analyses based on just two variables.

- The significance level (level of alpha). The default significance level is $\alpha = 0.05$ ($p \leq 0.05$; 1:20 chance that there is no difference or relationship between variables; see Chapter 9). It should be adjusted to a lower limit (often $\alpha = 0.01$) in order to avoid Type I error (spurious significant results) if a large number of statistical tests, such as correlations, are performed (see Chapter 9). However, the smaller the value of α, the larger the sample size needed to demonstrate a significant result.
- Directional (one-tailed) versus non-directional (two-tailed) test of probability. A non-directional (two-tailed) test of probability (Chapter 9) requires a much larger sample size to achieve significance compared to a directional (one-tailed) test.
- Response rate. Researchers are often wildly optimistic about the willingness of the public to engage in their survey. It is worth checking the response rate against those for similar types of study to see just how realistic their estimations were.

Chisholm et al. (2007)
There is no evidence that Chisholm et al. calculated a minimum sample size to be sure that they would detect significant predictors of adherence.
   The most complex analysis used was multiple regression, a multivariate test that included five independent (predictor) variables. Based on guidelines in Table 2.2, it would appear that a minimum of 100 sets of complete data (n) were needed. The authors acknowledge that their sample size of 65 was a limitation of their study, but this is no excuse as it should have been obvious at the planning stage.

Review notes:
Do the researchers give the criteria used to determine a minimum sample size? If not, does it look as if the sample size was likely to be adequate, using the information provided above?
What was the response rate and what might this say about the method of data collection used?
Do the researchers compare subgroups? If so, are the numbers likely to be large enough for statistical comparison?
Remember to look for the value of n in each set of statistical results. Does this indicate a high level of missing data, and is this likely to affect the reliability of the results?

Planned data analysis

The final part of the Method section usually reports:

- the type of statistical analysis used;
- checks on the distribution of the data, where appropriate;

- the significance level (level of alpha or value of p);
- the use of a one-tailed or two-tailed test of probability, unless this is stated with each set of results;
- the assumptions used to determine the sample size (if any).

Chisholm et al. (2007)
The following statistical tests were used to analyse the data:

- **Independent t test** (Chapter 11) to test for differences in diabetes knowledge scores between males and females.

- **One-way analysis of variance (ANOVA**; see Chapter 12) to test for differences in diabetes knowledge scores between social classes.

- **Correlation** (Pearson product-moment correlation, Chapter 15) to test for a relationship between diabetes knowledge and duration of diabetes.

- **Multiple regression** (Chapter 16) to test the combined ability of psycho-social variables to predict BGM frequency (measure of adherence).

Distribution of the data

All of the statistical tests listed above are 'parametric' tests, valid only if the outcome variable is continuous and approximates to the normal distribution. Therefore, the researchers must report on steps taken to ensure that the data conformed to the normal distribution. There are statistical tests for skewness (Chapter 4), but it is sufficient to report a visual inspection of the data. Data 'transformation' may be used to correct skewness, for example using logarithms or square roots.

Chisholm et al. (2007)
'Injection time variability' was reported not to conform to the normal distribution, so was 'transformed' to produce a normal distribution.

Inspections were also carried out to ensure that variables included in correlation and regression showed a linear relationship (see Chapter 15).

Significance level

Surveys often involve a lot of statistical tests on the same data, which increases the probability of Type I error (false significant result). To avoid this, the value of α may be adjusted to, say 0.02 (one in 50) or 0.01 (one in 100), depending on the number of tests conducted [$\alpha = 0.02$ implies $p \leq 0.02$].

> **Chisholm et al. (2007)**
> The significance level was set at $\alpha = 0.05$. However, a total of 17 variables were included and the tables of results included a total of *64* separate statistical tests, including a large number of correlations. A significance level of 0.05 (1:20) implies that 3 out of 60 results might achieve false significance – but which ones?

We would have suggested setting the significance level at $\alpha = 0.01$ (1:100) to eliminate the likelihood of one false significant result out of the 64 results reported. Dancey and Reidy (2007) recommend using the Bonferroni correction (divide the default significance level (0.05) by the number of tests). Many researchers regard this as too stringent. In this case, it would set the significance level at $0.05 \div 64$, i.e. $\alpha < 0.001$.

One- versus two-tailed test of probability

The strength and direction of the hypothesis determine whether a directional (one-tailed) or non-directional (two-tailed) test of probability[1] should be used (see Chapter 9). One-tailed probability implies that change or difference will occur in one direction only; two-tailed probability implies that change or difference may be in either direction. A one-tailed test is more likely to give a statistically significant result, but must only be used if adequately justified by the researcher.

> **Chisholm et al. (2007)**
> Chisholm et al. applied two-tailed tests of probability to their analyses, in keeping with their hypotheses. This is less susceptible to Type I error (false positive finding), but requires a larger sample size to avoid Type II error (false negative finding).

If the test of probability is not clearly stated in the Method or Results sections, it is a good idea to check the results to be sure that the appropriate test of probability was applied.

Review notes:
Did the researchers detail their planned statistical analyses, significance level and tests of probability?
Did they report on their inspections of the data to ensure that the assumptions or requirements for the planned statistical tests were adhered to?
Was the significance level appropriate to avoid (Type I error)? Was it adjusted to reflect the number of individual results reported? If not, how many results are 'at risk' of Type I error?

---

1 'Tail' refers to the tails or extreme ends of the distribution of the test results, see Chapter 9 for explanation.

Is the test of probability clearly identified in the Method or Results section? If a one-tailed test is used, is this adequately supported by theoretical or research-based evidence in the introduction?

Results

Survey results usually follow a typical pattern:

- **Descriptive statistics** (all types of survey). These summarise the distribution of each of the key variables.
- **Simple statistical tests of comparison and correlation** (social and epidemiological surveys).
- **Multivariate statistical tests** (most social and epidemiological surveys). The most common multivariate test is regression analysis, used to test which of several independent (predictor) variables predict a single, dependent (outcome) variable.

Descriptive statistics

These summarise the distribution of the variables and enable the reviewer to check the following:

1. Do the proportions in the data suggest any evidence of sample bias?

2. Is there any evidence of an odd or uneven distribution?

For more details, see Chapters 4 and 5.

Checking for sample bias

Do the proportions in the demographic data appear representative of the target population? Use your professional knowledge and, where necessary, check against reliable databases.

> **Chisholm et al. (2007)**
> This diabetic study included 42 boys and 23 girls. Does this reflect the proportion of boys to girls aged 2–8 years with type 1 diabetes in the general population?
>   The excess of diabetic boys in this study is high, and the researchers fail to account for this.

Check for non-normal distributions

If continuous data are analysed using parametric statistical tests (those that rely on the normal distribution), it is important to check that the data approximate to the normal distribution (see Chapter 4 for checks):

Chisholm et al. (2007)
Descriptive statistics are presented in the form of text:

Mean general knowledge of diabetes score was 76%, with a standard deviation (sd) of 12.44%.

The exact range of responses is not given, but we know that the maximum knowledge score possible is 100%. If a lot of people scored 100%, it might indicate the presence of a 'ceiling' effect, which could have skewed the data.

Assuming that the data conformed to the normal distribution (see Chapter 4), we can predict that approximately 95% of scores will be found in the range mean $\pm$ 2 sd. This would give 95% of scores on diabetic knowledge in the range

76% $\pm$ (2 $\times$ 12.44%) = 51% to 101%.

Given the approximation of 101% to the maximum possible score of 100%, the data would appear to approximate to the normal distribution with only slight evidence of skewness.

Mean injection frequency was documented as 7.9 (sd 1.94). Correcting these data to the nearest whole numbers, this finding indicates that 95% of all children received between 4 and 12 injections per day ($8 \pm 2 \times 2$), the average being 8 injections.

Chisholm et al. do not give the full range of values for each variable, but the formula (mean $\pm$ 2 sd) confirms that none of these extends much beyond the minimum or maximum values possible, thus confirming that the data appear to approximate to the normal distribution.

Review note:
Check the means and standard deviations to ensure that none of the distributions are seriously skewed. It they are, parametric tests of group difference, such as the t test or ANOVA, or tests of association such as Pearson correlation or multiple regression should not be used. Instead, the researchers should use nonparametric alternatives.

Statistical tests of comparison or group difference

It is quite common in surveys to compare subgroups within the sample, for example compare the health status of those living in different types of environment. The appropriate test of group difference depends on the type and distribution of the data, as indicated in Table 2.3.

Chisholm et al. (2007)
Chisholm et al. report under 'Data analysis' that *t* tests and ANOVA were used to compare groups on demographic, medical and psychosocial variables.

Table 2.3 Guide to selection of the appropriate test of group difference

Type of data for the dependent variable (the comparator)	Comparison between two independent groups*	Comparison between three or more independent groups*
Parametric: continuous data, normal distribution, similar standard deviations	Independent (unrelated) t test	One-way analysis of variance (known as ANOVA or F test)
Nonparametric: ordinal or non-normal continuous data	Mann–Whitney U test or signed rank test	Kruskal–Wallis ANOVA by ranks
Categorical data	Contingency analysis: Fisher exact probability (dichotomous data) or chi-square (χ^2)	Contingency analysis: chi-square (χ^2)

* These tests do not apply to paired data from matched samples or repeated measures taken from the same sample

Guided by Table 2.3, we can deduce that independent *t* tests (Chapter 11) were used to test for differences between boys and girls. One-way ANOVA (Chapter 12) was used to test for differences between socio-economic groups.

The assumptions of *t* tests and ANOVA are as follows:

- The dependent (outcome) variable is continuous and approximates to the normal distribution.
- The standard deviations for each group are approximately equal (this is referred to as homogeneity of variance).

Results normally include the value of the test statistic (*t* or *F* etc.), degrees of freedom (df) and the value of *p*. You will find examples of the presentation of these findings and their interpretation in Chapter 11.

Chisholm et al. (2007)
The researchers merely report finding no sex or social class differences on any of the variables measured. This suggests that further statistical tests were unlikely to be contaminated by sex or social class bias.

Review note:
Check that the assumptions for each statistical test of comparison have been met. Make a note of the results of these comparisons – you may need to take them into account when considering potential sources of bias in subsequent analyses.

Statistical tests of association (correlation)

It is usual to test for associations between key variables. Correlation measures the relationship between two continuous or ordinal variables taken from the same sample or group. Note, however, that a correlation between two variables does not imply a causal relationship between them (see Chapter 15).

There are two key assumptions to consider when reviewing tests of correlation:

- The association between the two variables must be linear (follow a straight line and not a curved or wavy line; see Chapter 15).

- Pearson correlation is a parametric test. It requires that both variables are continuous and neither is significantly skewed. If not, Spearman's rho (r_s), or Kendall's tau should be used.

When interpreting the results of correlation, there are three factors to take into account:

- the direction of the association (a minus sign indicates a negative association which means that an increase in one variable is associated with a decrease in the other);

- the strength of the association on a scale of 0 to ±1 (see Chapter 15 for interpretation);

- the statistical significance of the association.

Chisholm et al. (2007)

Better dietary knowledge was found to be associated with lower HbA1c levels ($r = -0.29$, $p < 0.03$).

$r = -0.29$ indicates that as dietary knowledge increased, HbA1c levels decreased; this is a weak negative association.

$p < 0.03$ indicates that this result is likely to be obtained less than once in 30 sets of observation if the null hypothesis is true and there really is *no* association between these variables.

This result is statistically significant since the value of p is less than the significance threshold of 0.05. But given that the researchers made more than 30 tests of correlation, Type I errors (false significance) are likely.

The researchers do not state if a one-tailed or two-tailed test of probability was used. Therefore, we checked the statistical tables for r to confirm the correct use of a non-directional (two-tailed) test, given the level of uncertainty described by the researchers in their aim and introduction.

Note that the researchers give no indication of the number (n) included in this analysis, so we had to assume that the data set was complete and all 65 participants completed the knowledge questionnaire in its entirety.

Multiple correlations are usually presented in the form of a correlation matrix which gives the correlation coefficient for each pair of variables. Significant associations are often identified using stars.

Chisholm et al. (2007)
An extract from the correlation matrix is given in Table 2.4. Note how the value of p gets smaller (more significant) as the value of r gets larger.

Table 2.4 Correlation matrix (based on data from Chisholm et al. 2007)

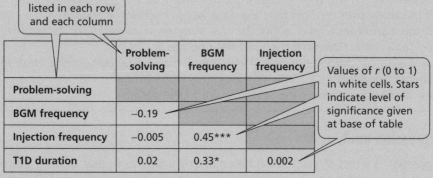

Each variable is listed in each row and each column

	Problem-solving	BGM frequency	Injection frequency
Problem-solving			
BGM frequency	−0.19		
Injection frequency	−0.005	0.45***	
T1D duration	0.02	0.33*	0.002

Values of r (0 to 1) in white cells. Stars indicate level of significance given at base of table

*2-tailed $p < 0.05$; **2-tailed $p < 0.01$; ***2-tailed $p < 0.001$ ($n = 65$)
(T1D = type 1 diabetes; BGM = blood glucose monitoring)

Using statistical tables, we noted that the critical value of r needed to achieve significance is just under 0.25, given $p \leq 0.05$ (two-tailed) and $n = 65$. Values of r closer to zero than ±0.25 show no significant association at this sample size.

The correlation matrix indicates no association between type 1 diabetes duration and injection frequency, or between type 1 diabetes duration and problem-solving, or between problem-solving and injection frequency.

Significant correlations were starred in the correlation matrix, the strongest being between the number of insulin injections given and frequency of BGM ($r = 0.45$, $p < 0.001$). $r = 0.45$ indicates a moderate association (the reviewer might wonder why it was not stronger). $p < 0.001$ (less than 1:1000) suggests that this finding is highly significant.

Correlations between psychosocial and diabetes-specific factors identify the following associations as significant ($p \leq 0.05$): 'family relationship maintenance' was associated with 'general knowledge about diabetes' ($r = 0.28$) and with 'non-milk extrinsic sugar (NMES) consumption' ($r = -0.39$), both weak to moderate associations.

It is noted that over 60 separate statistical analyses were reported, each with a significance level set at 0.05. This means that at least 3 results were susceptible to Type I error – but which ones?

Now review the values of p again using our recommended significance level of $\alpha = 0.01$, and the Bonferroni correction of $p \leq 0.001$. Using the Bonferroni correction, the only significant relationship is between frequency of BGM and the number of insulin injections given. But since these are both measures of diabetes treatment adherence and one often precedes the other, the relationship is hardly of interest in the context of the research aim.

Review notes:

Was the appropriate test of correlation (parametric or nonparametric) used, depending on the type and distribution of the data?

Did the researcher confirm that the data were checked for linearity?

Did the significance level allow for the number of correlations tested? How might a correction have changed the findings?

Was the test of probability clearly identified? If a one-tailed test was used, was this justified?

How might you interpret the relationships in the data?

Regression analysis

Regression is a test of association based on the assumption that there is a direct causal relationship between one or more predictor variables and a single outcome (dependent) variable. There are three main types of regression analysis:

1. **Simple linear regression** is a parametric test, similar to correlation, used where there is one continuous predictor variable and one continuous outcome variable (Chapter 15).

2. **Multiple regression** is used where there are several continuous or dichotomous predictor variables and one continuous outcome variable (Chapter 16).

3. **Logistic or loglinear regression** is used when the outcome variable is categorical, usually dichotomous (Chapter 16).

We explain and give examples of logistic regression in Chapter 1 (RCT) and focus here on multiple regression.

There are several important assumptions that underpin multiple regression (see Chapter 16). They should be confirmed by the researchers and verified, where possible, by the reviewer:

- Evidence is given to support a causal relationship between the predictor variables and the outcome variable.

- The relationships between the predictor and outcome variables are all linear (follow a straight line) and not curvilinear (form a curve).

- The outcome variable is continuous and conforms to the normal distribution.

- The predictor variables are either continuous or dichotomous.

- Predictor variables should be independent of each other (unrelated), so the correlation between them must not be high (we suggest no more than 0.7, though others suggest 0.8). High inter-correlations, referred to as collinearity or in the case of several variables 'multicollinearity', distort the analysis and results.

See chapter 16 for other complexities.

> **Chisholm et al. (2007)**
> Multiple regression was used to predict NMES intake, based on predictor variables selected because each demonstrated a significant correlation with NMES intake: carbohydrate knowledge, BGM frequency, age, family relationship maintenance.
>
> - No correlation between any pair of predictors was high, indicating an absence of multicollinearity.
> - Sugar consumption is a measure of adherence (to diet) specified in the aim, and is therefore an appropriate outcome variable.
> - BGM frequency sits very oddly as a predictor variable because, using the researcher's own theoretical perspective, it is also a measure of adherence (to diabetes treatment regime).

Multiple regression analysis includes one variable at a time until no additional predictor adds significantly to the amount of variance explained by the regression model (see Chapter 16 for an explanation of the procedure).

The results of multiple regression are usually given in the form of a table that ideally includes certain key information, as illustrated in Table 2.5.

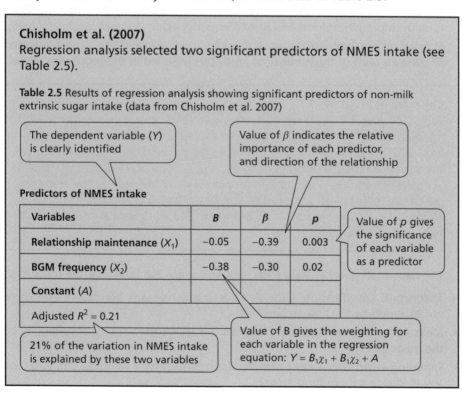

Chisholm et al. (2007)
Regression analysis selected two significant predictors of NMES intake (see Table 2.5).

Table 2.5 Results of regression analysis showing significant predictors of non-milk extrinsic sugar intake (data from Chisholm et al. 2007)

The dependent variable (Y) is clearly identified

Value of β indicates the relative importance of each predictor, and direction of the relationship

Predictors of NMES intake

Variables	B	β	p
Relationship maintenance (X_1)	−0.05	−0.39	0.003
BGM frequency (X_2)	−0.38	−0.30	0.02
Constant (A)			
Adjusted $R^2 = 0.21$			

Value of p gives the significance of each variable as a predictor

21% of the variation in NMES intake is explained by these two variables

Value of B gives the weighting for each variable in the regression equation: $Y = B_1 \chi_1 + B_1 \chi_2 + A$

The multiple regression model consists of a straight line equation:

$Y = B_1X_1 + B_2X_2 + \ldots + \text{constant}$.

In this equation:

Y is the value of the outcome variable (NMES consumption);
X_1, X_2, etc. are the values for each predictor variable;
B_1, B_2, etc. are the weightings applied to each predictor variable (each is measured using a different scale, so these values have no interpretive meaning).

Chisholm et al. do not include the value of a constant, so their regression equation is incomplete. Had it been included, NMES consumption for an individual child diabetes patient would be predicted by the following equation:

(-0.05 × their score on relationship maintenance) + (-0.38 × their score on BGM frequency) + (the value of the constant).

Note that the values of B need to be accompanied by 95% confidence intervals for application in practice. This would indicate the range of NMES consumption scores likely to contain the true value 95% of the time.
The table of results also includes β, p and R^2.

β measures the relative importance of each predictor variable. Table 2.5 indicates that relationship maintenance ($\beta = 0.39$) is a slightly more important predictor of NMES intake than BGM frequency ($\beta = 0.3$).

p gives the probability that each predictor contributes to the outcome. Both relationship maintenance and BGM frequency achieve significance ($p < 0.05$).

R^2 measures the combined power of the predictors to explain the outcome. Adjusted R^2 takes account of the number of predictors included in the regression model.

Chisholm et al. (2007)
Table 2.5 gives $R^2 = 0.21$, which means that 'relationship maintenance' and 'blood glucose monitoring' combine to explain 21% of the variance associated with adherence, measured using sugar intake. The remaining 79% of the variance remains unexplained.

These results might be more impressive if there was good reason to suppose that there might be a causal link between BGM and sugar intake. It makes little logical sense if both are identified as measures of adherence to diabetic management.

The value of R^2 rarely exceeds 60%. Reasons for low values include the following:

- **Theoretical specification error**. Are there any relevant predictors that were not included by the researchers?
- **Measurement error**. Are there reasons to suspect the validity or reliability of the measures used?
- **Sampling error**. This is most likely in small convenience samples. Can you spot any evidence of sampling error?

Review notes:
Check that the researchers have adhered to all the assumptions of multiple regression:

- *The type of data and distribution are appropriate.*
- *The associations between each predictor and the outcome variable have been checked for linearity and, where necessary, the data are transformed to assure this (see Chapter 15).*
- *The significance level is adjusted for the number of correlations tested.*
- *The test of probability, if one-tailed, is justified.*
- *Causal relationship between the independent (predictor) variables and the dependent (outcome) variable are justified.*
- *There is no strong correlation between any of the predictor variables (termed 'multicollinearity').*

What do the results mean?
How much of the variance is accounted for by the regression model?
Can you think of any reasons why the R^2 value is not higher?

Conclusions from our survey review

If you have recorded review notes, compare your appraisal of the Chisholm et al. survey with our ideas below.

Chisholm et al. (2007)
The study poses an important research question for practice, but is subject to a number of serious limitations:

- It was based on a convenience sample in a single location which may challenge the generalisability of the findings.
- There is doubt about the validity and reliability of some of the measures used.
- The significance level (two-tailed $p \leq 0.05$) needed to be adjusted to a more stringent level to allow for the large number of statistical tests of correlation included in the study. However, this would have required a larger sample size to avoid Type II error.
- In any event, the sample size was too small to produce reliable results using multivariate analysis.
- Blood glucose monitoring frequency was treated as a predictor of adherence, even though it is also a measure of adherence.

Overall, we would have to conclude that the sample size was inadequate and the findings theoretically and statistically weak.

PART 2
INTERPRETING STATISTICAL CONCEPTS

This part of the book focuses on factors that determine the type of statistics used to analyse quantitative data (Figure P2.1), as well as factors that influence the interpretation of the statistical results (Figure P2.2).

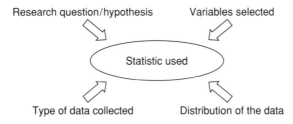

Figure P2.1 Factors that determine the statistical analysis used

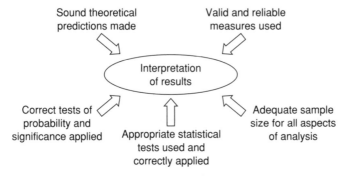

Figure P2.2 Factors that influence the interpretation of the statistical results

Each chapter addresses a specific set of questions that you may have and explains key aspects of each factor, illustrated with worked examples. As most of these concepts are interlinked, it is not possible to present them in a sequence that makes complete sense from a learning perspective and it will be necessary to cross-reference between chapters.

If you answer 'no' to any of the questions in Figure P2.3, we suggest that you read the appropriate chapter. If you answer 'yes' to the following questions, use Part 3 to refresh your memory as needed.

I am familiar with the different types of data (continuous, ordinal, categorical).

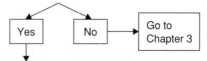

I understand the concept of the normal distribution and how to interpret mean and standard deviation. I can tell from descriptive statistics if the data are skewed.

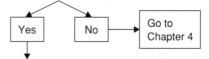

I understand how to interpret median and percentiles and can 'visualise' data given in the form of tables.

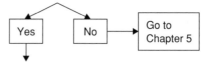

I am familiar with the statistical methods of establishing the validity and reliability when measuring health concepts.

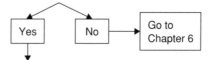

I understand the concept of random sampling and how a non-probability sample can affect the generalisability of research findings.

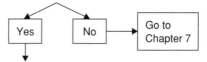

I am able to judge if a sample size is adequate, based on the type and distribution of the data, and the statistical tests used. I understand the meaning of 'intention-to-treat' analysis.

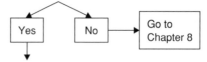

I am familiar with the meaning of one-tailed and two-tailed tests and p-values and know how to judge if the correct test of probability has been applied.

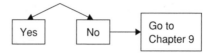

Figure P2.3 Statistical knowledge check

3 Measuring Variables:
Continuous, Ordinal and Categorical Data

KEY QUESTIONS

- What is meant by the term 'variable'?
- What types of measurement scale are used in research?
- What is the difference between continuous, ordinal and categorical data?
- What impact do these types of data have on statistical analysis?

Introduction

This chapter focuses on the identification of variables and types of measurement used.

BASIC TERMS
Variable is measureable characteristic, so called because measurements vary between individuals, across time and/or according to different sets of conditions or influences.
Data refers to a set of measurements.

What is meant by a 'variable'?

A variable is a measurable concept that represents or characterises an object, person, environment or circumstance. The concept must be clearly defined and measured using a valid and reliable measurement scale.

It is useful to separate the concept from the form of measurement:

- The concept forms the basis of the hypothesis, which needs to be justified in the Introduction section.
- The selection of an appropriate measure is presented and/or justified in the Method section.

For example:

- Temperature is a concept.
- The Celsius, Fahrenheit and Kelvin scales are all measures of temperature.

Independent and dependent variables

Quantitative research is commonly based on theoretical predictions known as hypotheses. For example, the researcher predicts that a particular event or outcome is associated with a particular set of circumstances.

Variables measure both the effect or outcome (the dependent variable) and its causes or predictors (the independent variables).

It is helpful when critiquing a piece of research to make a note of the concepts referred to in the Introduction and to distinguish between causal factors (the independent variables) and effects (the dependent variables). The next step is to look in the Method section to identify how each of these variables was measured.

Example

Ilhan et al. (2008) conducted a survey of 474 female nurses working at a university hospital in Turkey in order to study the extent of burnout. Their hypothesis was that a combination of nurse characteristics and working conditions contribute as causal factors. They measured the following variables:

Dependent variables

Concepts	Measurement
Burnout	Maslach Burnout Inventory (Turkish translation), 22 items
Three subscales of burnout, as indicated by the scale names:	Emotional Exhaustion (EE) scale
	Depersonalization (DP) scale
	Personal Accomplishment (PA) scale

Independent variables

Concepts	Measurement
Age	Years
Nursing experience	Years in nursing
Workload	Daily working hours Weekly working hours
Nursing specialty	Medical/surgical
Work satisfaction	Measurements based on various aspects of work

Measurement scales

Three basic types of measurement scale determine the type of data used in research:

1. **Continuous (interval) data** are based a scale of magnitude that has equidistant intervals between each point on the scale (e.g. a score of 0–10; blood pressure in millimetres of mercury, height in inches).

2. **Ordinal data** are measured using a scale that has at least four points numbered sequentially in ascending or descending order. These are not necessarily separated by equal intervals, as in the four-point Likert scale, where 1 stands for 'strongly agree', 2 for 'agree', 3 for 'disagree' and 4 for 'strongly disagree'.

3. **Categorical (nominal) data** can be assigned to categories that may be given numbers for the purpose of analysis but which have no meaningful numerical relationship. Examples include ethnic groups or professional grades. Categorical data that consist of only two categories are referred to as **dichotomous** (e.g. sex, male (1) or female (2); response, yes (1) or no (0)).

The Ilhan et al. study included all three different types of data:

Continuous data

- Age, in years
- Length of time in the profession, in years
- Daily work duration, in hours
- Weekly working hours, in hours
- Scores on each subscale of the Maslach Burnout Inventory

Ordinal data

- Satisfaction was originally measured using a series of five-point rating scales. However, nobody recorded a response using the mid-point, effectively turning this measure into a four-point scale.

Categorical data

- Nursing specialty: surgical/medical

Example

Note that the slightly unequal intervals in single verbal rating scales tend to be ironed out when several items are added together, as in the Maslach Burnout Inventory and many other quality of life questionnaires. Therefore, scores on these scales are usually treated as continuous data.

The Maslach Burnout Inventory, used in the Ilhan et al. study, consists of 22 items, each measured using a five-point verbal rating scale (scored 0–4). These items are grouped into three subscales. Scores on items within each subscale are added to give a single continuous score. For example, the Emotional Exhaustion scale contains nine items and gives a score of between 0 and 36 which is treated as continuous.

Example

Why is it best to collect continuous data wherever possible?

Continuous data provide rich information. When used as a dependent variable, they make it possible to detect a small change. Therefore the statistical tests based on a continuous dependent variable are more powerful and require a smaller sample size to achieve a statistically significant result (assuming there is one to be found).

Continuous data can, once collected, be grouped to form an ordinal or categorical variable if required for practical reasons. Take the example of age:

- Age in years (continuous data). This measurement has good ability to detect small differences or changes and may be analysed using the most powerful parametric statistics (see Chapter 4). The data may be grouped to facilitate age group comparisons, if required.

- Age in five groups: 22–26, 27–31, 32–36, 37–41, 42+ (ordinal data). This form of measurement is less sensitive and has less flexibility in terms of data analysis, necessitating less powerful nonparametric statistics (see Chapter 5).

- Age in two groups: under 40, 40 or over (dichotomous data). Categorical or dichotomous data form the essential basis for group comparisons, but are insensitive when used as a form of measurement scale (see Chapter 5).

This type of data is normally treated as ordinal provided there are at least four scale points. Data based on only three scale points (for example yes, don't know, no) are normally treated as categorical.

Example

Janssen et al. (2004) recorded weight using a continuous scale. But in order to compare the characteristics of those in different weight categories, Janssen et al. divided their sample into three discrete categories: normal weight, overweight and obese. Their sample size of 15,000 ensured adequate numbers in each weight group for the purposes of comparison.

Ilhan et al. dichotomised some variables following data collection, for ease of interpretation: weekly working hours (up to 8 hours, more than 8 hours); workload (heavy, not heavy); and work satisfaction (satisfied, not satisfied). It might have been difficult for individuals to respond in such a black-and-white way, so it made sense to categorise the data after data collection.

Each time data are categorised unnecessarily, sensitivity is lost, data analysis is constrained and a larger sample size may be required for the analysis. Those conducting small-scale studies are unwise to collect continuous data, such as age, in a categorised form unless it is likely to lead to a high rate of missing data or attrition, for example if participants are unwilling to give personal details. Large-scale surveys often categorise or reduce data, such as age, into two or three categories so that it is easier to interpret them and make direct comparisons, but this approach is not really suitable for small-scale studies.

Summary

- Variables are measured using one of three basic types of measurement scale: continuous (interval), ordinal and categorical (nominal).

- Continuous data are (subject to fulfilling certain assumptions) described and analysed using the most powerful parametric statistics.

- Other types of data are analysed using nonparametric statistics.

- Each time data is grouped into a smaller number of categories, information is lost and a larger sample size is required to identify a statistically significant result.

4 Describing Continuous Data:
The Normal Distribution

KEY QUESTIONS

- What is meant by 'descriptive statistics'?
- What is meant by the 'normal distribution' and why is it so important?
- What is meant by the term 'parametric'?
- What information do the mean and standard deviation really convey?
- How can I tell if the data conform to the normal distribution?
- What is the relationship between standard deviation, value of p (probability) and the normal distribution?

Introduction: descriptive statistics

Only researchers have access to the full set of 'raw' data. 'Descriptive statistics' are a statistical shorthand for a description or summary of numerical data for the benefit of the reader or reviewer.

In quantitative research, data are sometimes referred to by statisticians as 'qualitative data'. This simply means 'descriptive data' and must *not* be confused with the same term when used in qualitative research.

Chapter 3 identified three basic types of data: **categorical**, **ordinal** and **continuous**. Each of these types of data has its own set of descriptive statistics. Once you become familiar with these, you will be able to 'picture' patterns in data and spot anomalies or inconsistencies that are useful when critiquing the data analysis and research findings.

In this chapter, we focus on statistics used to describe continuous data and their relationship to the normal distribution.

BASIC TERMS
Value refers to a recorded measurement.
Distribution refers to the pattern of values recorded for a particular variable.

The normal distribution

The normal distribution is a ubiquitous feature of the natural world. Most naturally occurring variables measured using a continuous scale demonstrate a bell-shaped symmetrical pattern, with most values lying close to the mean (average) and few values lying towards each extreme end of the range. This pattern of variation is termed the 'normal distribution'.

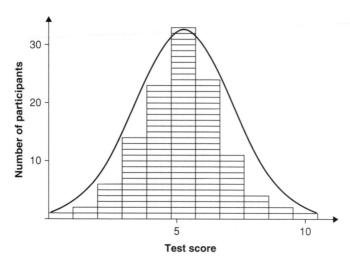

Figure 4.1 Histogram illustrating approximation of data set to the normal distribution, with overlay of the normal distribution curve

The normal distribution forms the basis of parametric statistics, which are based on the geometric properties of the normal distribution curve.

Researchers are able to check the shape of the distribution for each variable by plotting a histogram (continuous form of bar chart), as in Figure 4.1 where test scores are plotted against the number of participants who recorded each value.

In Figure 4.1, the range of possible scores for this variable is from 0 to 10. Out of the total of 112 participants, only two participants scored either 0 or 10. The majority scored between 4 and 6.

Shoe size is a useful small group exercise to familiarise yourself with the concept of the normal distribution. You need about 20 people, preferably of the same gender.

1. First find those with the largest and the smallest sizes in the group to establish the range.

2. Towards the bottom of a whiteboard or large piece of paper, draw a horizontal line and label with all sizes in the range, including half sizes.

3. Fill in the graph by going round the group and adding a block for each person in the appropriate size column – as in the example in Figure 4.2, which was designed for females.

4. If you have males and females, use a different coloured pen for each sex.

Figure 4.2 illustrates how the distinctive bell-shaped distribution gradually emerges as observations are added. If the class is mixed sex, the range of sizes will be greater. If the class has an imbalance of men and women, the distribution will no longer appear to conform to the normal distribution as large male or small female 'outliers' distort the pattern of distribution. If you used different coloured pens for each sex, you should see two separate distributions emerge.

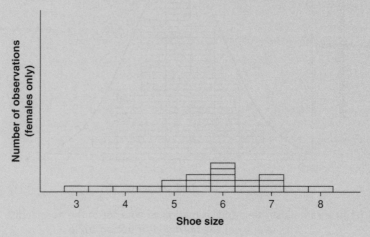

Figure 4.2 Histogram of women's shoe size

Variables rarely demonstrate a smooth normal curve, even when taken from a huge population. Thus data are usually described as 'approximating' to the normal distribution. It is difficult to assume that data approximate to the normal distribution if the data set is small (less than 30).

Example

In Table 4.1, height measurements, taken from a sample of nearly 1 million healthy Swedish adult men (Magnussen et al. 2006), show good approximation to the normal distribution. This is easier to appreciate then presented in the form of a bar chart, as in Figure 4.3.

Table 4.1 Table of distribution of height measurements (from Magnussen et al. 2006)

Height (cm)	*N* (number of cases)	%
<165	10,176	1.1
165–169	49,734	5.2
170–174	161,340	17.0
175–179	273,846	28.8
180–184	260,394	27.4
185–189	140,700	14.8
190–194	44,961	4.7
>195	10,068	1.1

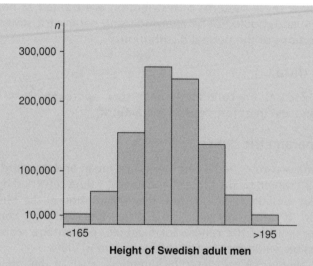

Figure 4.3 Bar chart showing height distributions from Table 4.1

Deviations from the normal distribution may be due to artificial distortion within a population. For example, if medical interventions keep people alive who would otherwise have died, this will bias the age distribution. A non-normal distribution can also indicate sampling bias, so checking the distribution is an important review task.

Non-normal distributions

There are three types of non-normal distribution to look for (see Figure 4.4):

- A **skewed** distribution is where the measurements are biased towards one end of the distribution.

- A **peaked** distribution occurs where there is little variation in the data (Kurtosis), as illustrated in Figure 4.4, or a very flat distribution.

- A **multimodal** distribution is where there is more than one commonly occurring value (mode). **Bimodal** refers to two commonly occurring values. These can only be detected on inspection of a bar chart or histogram, so the reviewer is reliant on the researcher to detect and report this.

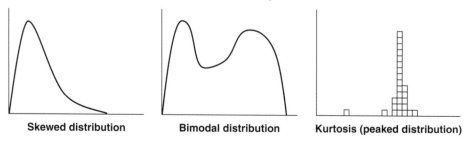

Figure 4.4 Three types of non-normal distribution

Data that follow these patterns of distribution are treated as nonparametric (see Chapter 5) and should not be analysed using parametric statistics that rely on the assumptions of the normal distribution.

Parametric data

This chapter focuses on continuous data that approximate to the normal distribution and are therefore termed 'parametric'.

Describing parametric data

Parametric data are described using the range, mean and standard deviation.

The **range** is marked by the highest and lowest values recorded by the sample for a particular variable. You may find this information in the Method or the Results section. If not, apply your professional knowledge or common sense to predict the limits of the range. For example, percentage scores imply the minimum possible value is zero and the maximum is 100%.

The **mean** (average) is calculated by summing up all of the individual scores and dividing by the total number of subjects, as in the example in Table 4.2.

Example

Table 4.2 illustrates shoe size measurements taken from a total of 21 women (i.e. $n = 21$).

Table 4.2 Table of shoe sizes

Number of subjects (n)	Shoe size	Row totals (n × size)
1	3	3
1	4	4
1	4.5	4.5
2	5	10
3	5.5	16.5
5	6	30
2	6.5	13
3	7	21
1	7.5	7.5
1	8	8
1	9	9
$n = 21$		Sum (Σ) = 126.5
Mean shoe size = 126.5 ÷ 21 = 6.02		

In the normal distribution, the mean value lies roughly half-way between the highest and lowest values in the range.

The **standard deviation** is a measure of spread or variation of values around the mean, assuming the variable conforms to the normal distribution. It is measured as distance from the mean using the original units of measurement, as illustrated in Figure 4.5 using an example of shoe size in which the standard deviation is calculated to be 1.0 shoe sizes. The reviewer does not need to calculate standard deviation, but the formula helps to understand the concept.

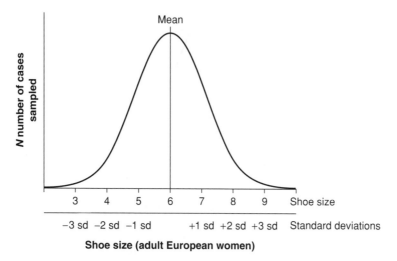

Figure 4.5 Distribution of women's shoe sizes with a standard deviation of 1 shoe size

---

Standard Deviation

The formula for the standard deviation is:

$$\sqrt{\frac{\Sigma(X-\text{mean})^2}{n-1}}$$

where X represents each individual value, Σ means sum, and n is the sample size. It helps to break down this formula into stages:

1. The mean is subtracted from each recorded value and the result squared.
2. All of the squared values are added together and the sum is divided by sample size minus one ($n - 1$), which is called the degrees of freedom (which statisticians use in preference to the sample size as a precaution against overestimation). This gives a measure known as the 'variance'.
3. The square root of the variance is the standard deviation.

The standard deviation is a standardised measure, which means that it has certain constant properties, based on the normal distribution curve, which we explain next.

Properties of the normal distribution curve

Approximately 68% of a given population will record a value or score within the range of values determined by (mean ± 1 standard deviation), referred to as within one standard deviation of the mean (Figure 4.6).

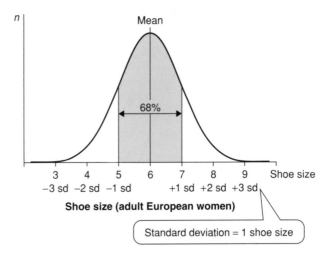

Figure 4.6 Normal distribution showing the proportion of the population whose shoe sizes are within one standard deviation of the mean (mean ± 1 sd)

Approximately 95% of a given population will record a score that is within the range of values determined by (mean ± 2 standard deviations), as shown in Figure 4.7.[1]

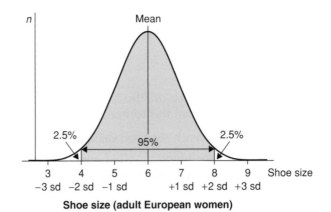

Figure 4.7 Normal distribution showing the proportion of the population whose show sizes are within two standard deviations of the mean

---

1 The actual figure is (mean ± 1.96 sd) but an approximation is adequate for review purposes.

These proportions under the normal distribution curve provide the basis of probability (p values).

Standard deviation and probability

In the shoe size example, where the female population mean is 6 and the standard deviation is 1, approximately 95% of values lie within 2 standard deviations (i.e. 2 shoe sizes) of the mean, thus between 4 and 8. This interval, 4–8, defines the 95% confidence interval (CI) for women's shoe size. This range of shoe sizes will predict correct women's shoe size about 95% of the time.

It also implies that less than 5% of values fall outside this range ($p \leq 0.05$). These 5% are the unlikely values, labelled statistically significant, that fall within the two extreme 'tails' of the normal distribution. Hence the origin of the terms one-tailed and two-tailed probability (see Chapter 9).

Full descriptive statistics from the data on shoe size might read:

Based on findings from a sample of European women, mean shoe size is 6 (sd 1; range 2–10; 95% CI 4–8)

This implies that:

- The average women's shoe size is 6.
- The standard deviation is 1 shoe size.
- Shoe sizes range between 2 and 10.
- The 95% confidence interval is 4–8.

Example

How can I tell if a set of data approximate to the normal distribution?

The concept of standard deviation only makes sense if the data approximate to the normal distribution. The reviewer should look for the following **clues to skewness** in the descriptive statistics for each variable, at the beginning of the Results section:

1. The mean is located well towards one end of the distribution (i.e. close to the highest or lowest recorded value).
2. A tendency to skewness is indicated if the calculation (mean ± 2 sd) lies beyond the highest or lowest value recorded for the sample, or outside the range of values possible on the measurement scale used.
3. Skewness is certain if the calculation (mean ± 1 sd) lies beyond the highest or lowest value recorded for the sample, or outside the range of values possible on the measurement scale used.
4. If values for both mean and median are given and if the median is significantly different from the mean, the data are skewed. We explain this after the following example.

Holland et al. (2005) studied post-discharge care for elderly people. Baseline measurements were reported as:

Mean (sd) length of stay in days = 13.6 (14.6); n = 437.

The authors fail to give the range of stay, but we can calculate that:

Mean $\pm$ 2 sd = 13.6 $\pm$ (2 × 14.6) = −15.6 to 42.8 days.

Length of stay cannot be less than 0 days, so these data must be skewed. In Figure 4.8, we have constructed a bar chart, based on our assumption of what might be happening.

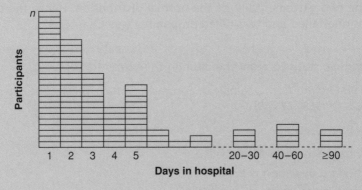

Figure 4.8 Bar chart showing likely skewed distribution of length of hospital stay

You can see that it is fairly meaningless to give average stay as 13.6 days. We deal with descriptive statistics for skewed distributions in Chapter 5. In this case, the median would have been a better indicator of average stay. From looking at the data, we estimate that this would be in the region of 3 days. Mean average has been distorted by 'outliers' who had an extended stay.

Relationship of the mean to the median

The median is the middle value when all of the collected values are placed in ascending (rank) order. If the data conform to the normal distribution, the mean is equal to the median (and the mode, which is the most commonly occurring value). In a skewed distribution, the mean and median are separated, as illustrated in Figure 4.9.

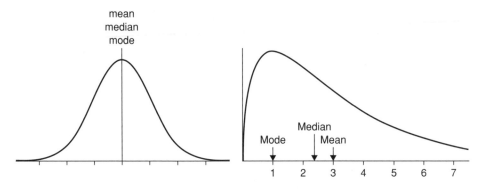

Figure 4.9 Comparison of features of normal and skewed distributions

Table 4.3 illustrates the position of the median value in the distribution of shoe size measurements.

Table 4.3 Distribution of shoe size measurements, showing the median

n	size	Total (n × size)
1	3	3
1	4	4
1	4.5	4.5
2	5	10
3	5.5	16.5
5	6	30
2	6.5	13
3	7	21
1	7.5	7.5
1	8	8
1	9	9
n = 21		126.5
Mean = 126.5/21		6.02

Middle value (median) ⟹ (row with n = 5, size 6)

If we lined up all the individuals in order of shoe size, the shoe size of the middle person would be the median.

The results give a median of 6 and a mean of 6.02. Since the mean and median are almost exactly equal, the data are not skewed.

Example

Unfortunately, it is rare for the researchers to give both the mean and the median. However, the researchers may report a statistical test for skewness, based on this difference, to demonstrate that their data conform to the normal distribution. If

$$\frac{\text{mean} - \text{median}}{\text{sd}} > 0.2$$

that is, if the mean minus the median, divided by the standard deviation, gives a value greater than 0.2, then skewness is evident.

Example

Table 4.4 Descriptive statistics (from Ilhan et al. 2008)

	Mean (sd)	Median
Duration in the profession (years)	9.4 (5.7)	8
Daily work duration (hours)	9.2 (2.4)	8
Weekly work duration (hours)	41.7 (5.5)	40

An extract from the descriptive statistics given in Ilhan et al. (2008) is given in Table 4.4. Applying the formula to test for skewness, we have:

for duration of profession

$$\frac{9.4 - 8}{5.7} = 0.175 \qquad \text{(not skewed)};$$

for daily work duration

$$\frac{9.2 - 8}{2.4} = 0.5 \qquad \text{(severely skewed)};$$

and for weekly work duration

$$\frac{41.7 - 40}{5.5} = 0.3 \qquad \text{(skewed)}.$$

The conclusion is as follows:

- Data for duration in the profession conform to the normal distribution and meet the assumptions for parametric statistics
- Data for daily and weekly work duration appear to be skewed and may violate the assumptions for parametric statistics

Researchers are expected to report on the steps they have taken to ensure that continuous data approximate to the normal distribution before using parametric statistics to analyse the data.

Summary

- Properties of the normal distribution curve mean that approximately 95% of observations lie within ± 2 standard deviations of the mean.
- $p \leq 0.05$ refers to the 5% of unusual values that lie in the extreme 'tails' of the normal distribution.
- If the data are skewed, parametric statistics should not be used.

5 Describing Nonparametric Data

KEY QUESTIONS

KEY QUESTIONS

- What is meant by the term 'nonparametric'?
- What is conveyed by the terms 'median' and 'percentile'?
- What is meant by rank order?
- What is the difference between parametric and nonparametric statistics?

Introduction

In this chapter we explain what is meant by nonparametric data, together with the descriptive statistics that are used to summarise continuous (interval) data that *do not* conform to the normal distribution, ordinal data and categorical (nominal) data. For explanations of the different types of data, refer back to Chapter 3.

BASIC TERMS

Nonparametric refers to ordinal or categorical data and continuous data that do not conform to the normal distribution. It is also used to describe the statistics used to analyse these types of data.

Rank order refers to the numerical rank position of each value, once all of the values are placed in ascending order.

Describing data that are non-normal or ordinal

The following terms are used to describe continuous data that do not approximate to the normal distribution, and ordinal data:

- The **range** is indicated by the highest and lowest recorded values.
- The **median** is the middle value. When the scores from each individual are set out in order of value, the median is the score in the middle.
- A **percentile** refers to the percentage of the population whose scores lie below the value given.
- The **quartiles** are the values that demark the highest or lowest 25% of the sample or population.
- The **interquartile range** is a nonparametric measure of spread in the data that gives the range of measurements for the 50% of the population whose values lie between the 25th and the 75th percentile.

What is the median and what is meant by 'rank order'?

The median is illustrated using the following example of shoe size.

Take a group of 16 women lined up in order of their shoe size and then allocated a rank position based on their shoe size, as illustrated in Table 5.1.

Table 5.1 Illustration of rank positions used in nonparametric statistics

Median
↓

Individuals	1	2	3	4	5	6	7	8	9	10	11	12	13	14	15	16
Shoe sizes	3	4	5	5	5	6	6	6	6	6	6	6	7	7	7	9
Rank position	1	2	4	4	4	9	9	9	9	9	9	9	14	14	14	16

Shared rank positions

The rank position relates to the position of the individual in the hierarchy. But, unlike positions in a race, statistical ranking takes account of ties when assigning the rank position. For example, size 5 is taken by individuals 3, 4 and 5, thus sharing the rank position of 4. Size 6 is taken by individuals 6 to 12 who therefore share the rank of 9. And so on.

The median is found between individuals 8 and 9 who share a rank position of 9. Thus the median value is 9.

You might note from the above example that it makes no difference to the median if the person with the largest size feet takes size 9 or size 14. There are only 16 possible rank positions, so the maximum rank position of the person with the largest feet is 16.

Nonparametric statistics are based on these rank positions and not on the actual values. This corrects for skewness, outliers and other odd distributions, as well as unequal intervals between points on a scale, as in ordinal data.

Percentiles

Each percentile represents values for the percentage of the population ranked below that value. Thus the 3rd percentile is the value such that 3% of the sample/population lie below it, and the 10th percentile is the value such that 10% of the sample/population lie below it (also referred to as the lowest **decile**). The 25th percentile is also called the **lower quartile** or **first quartile**, while the 75th quartile is also called the **upper quartile** or **third quartile**. The 50th percentile is more commonly called the median.

Example

Epidemiological data indicate that, at the age of 20 months, percentiles for a male child's weight are as follows:

- 3rd percentile = 22 lb. A child who weighs less than 22 lb at the age of 2 years is described as being below the 3rd percentile, meaning the child is among the lowest 3% for their age in terms of weight.
- 50th percentile = 26.75 lb. A child who weighs 26.75 lb is on the 50th percentile and therefore the median weight for their age.
- 97th percentile = 33 lb. A child who weighs more than 33 lb at that age is above the 97th percentile and is among the heaviest 3% for their age.

The **interquartile range** gives the range of values for the 50% of the population whose measurements lie between the lower and upper quartiles.

Descriptive statistics from Ilhan et al. (2008) for continuous but skewed data are given in Table 5.2. These data tell us that in terms of duration in the profession: 50% have been in the profession for between 5 and 12 years, with a median of 8 years; 25% of the sample have been in the profession for less than 5 years; 25% have been in the profession for more than 12 years.

Table 5.2 Nonparametric descriptive statistics (from Ilhan et al. 2008)

	Median	Interquartile range
Duration in the profession (years)	8	5–12
Daily work duration (hours)	8	8–9
Weekly work duration (hours)	40	40–44

Bar charts

Bar charts are often used to provide a visual representation of ordinal data. They are easier to read than tables and there is nothing to prevent the reviewer from constructing their own if it helps to understand the data. We have illustrated this in Figure 5.1.

It is good to see as much information as possible in a single bar chart. Proportions or percentages are more informative than raw values, provided the sample size is large enough for this to make sense (at least 30).

The bar chart in Figure 5.1 is based on data provided in a table of results. Note that the age categories are treated as ordinal data. The bar chart conveys the same information but is more easily understood. It takes up valuable space and is therefore only usually used in descriptive surveys.

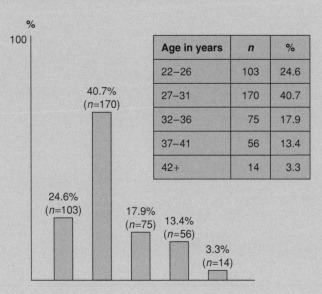

Age in years	n	%
22–26	103	24.6
27–31	170	40.7
32–36	75	17.9
37–41	56	13.4
42+	14	3.3

Figure 5.1 Bar chart of age data (based on data from Ilhan et al. 2008)

Describing categorical (nominal) data

Categorical data are described as numbers and percentages, commonly in the form of a table.

Ilhan et al. (2008) gave details of work conditions using numbers and percentages (see Table 5.3).

Table 5.3 Table of categorical results (from Ilhan et al. 2008)

Weekly work duration	n	%
≤ 40 hours	296	70.8
> 40 hours	122	27.2

Percentages provide more useful information than raw numbers provided the sample size is sufficiently large – it makes no sense to give percentages if there are less than 20–30 observations.

Categorical data has visual impact when presented using a pie chart (see Figure 5.2), though these are usually only used when these data are of primary importance, as in a market-type survey.

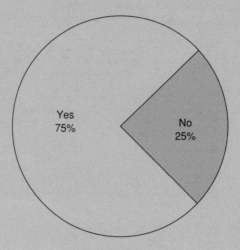

Figure 5.2 Pie chart

Summary

- Ordinal data and interval data that do not approximate to the normal distribution are described and analysed using nonparametric statistics, based on rank order.
- The median is used instead of the mean to describe the mid-point of scaled nonparametric data.
- Categorical data are summarised using percentages.

Further reading

Pett, M.A. (1997) *Nonparametric Statistics for Health Care Research: Statistics for Small Samples and Unusual Distributions*. Thousands Oaks, CA: Sage.

Siegel, S. and Castellan, N.J. (1988) *Nonparametric Statistics for the Behavioral Sciences* (second edition). New York: McGraw-Hill.

6 Measuring Concepts:
Validity and Reliability

KEY QUESTIONS

- What statistical criteria are used to judge validity and reliability?
- How should reliability scores be interpreted?

Introduction

Many variables, such as quality of life and pain, are abstract concepts for which measurement scales must be constructed. Statistics cannot compensate for methods of measurement that are either invalid or unreliable.

In this chapter, we explain some statistical procedures used to test for validity and reliability.

BASIC TERMS

Validity: A valid measure is one that accurately represents the concept or construct that it is intended to measure.

Reliability: A reliable measure is one that consistently gives the same measurement when used in the same or comparable conditions.

Tests of validity

Variables such as depression, burnout and quality of life are measured using a self-report scale, which is often made up of responses to a series of individual items:

- Each item is represented by an individual question or statement to which the response is measured using a verbal rating scale, such as a Likert scale (see Chapter 3).
- Responses are added together to give an overall score on composite scale or dimension that has a meaningful label attached to it.

There are several different ways of judging the validity of the resulting scale, some of which involve statistical testing. They include:

- **Face validity** – does it look right? This is based on professional judgement.
- **Content validity** – do the items accurately represent all aspects of the concept? This is informed by theory and based on judgement.
- **Construct validity** – how well does the measure represent the concept at a theoretical level? This is confirmed using factor analysis.

- **Predictive validity** (criterion validity) – how well does the measure predict real life outcomes or effects? This is measurable against an independent clinical measure.

- **Concurrent validity** – how well does the measure correlate with existing measures of the same concept? This is measurable against an alternative valid measure.

Only construct, predictive and concurrent validity are measurable.

Construct validity

This is best illustrated using an example. The health belief model, widely used as a predictor of health outcomes, is based on four separate dimensions:

- perceived vulnerability (to a disease);

- perceived severity (of the disease);

- perceived benefits (of taking preventive action);

- perceived barriers (to taking preventive action).

The most common methods of confirming the structure of these scales are factor analysis and principal components analysis.[1]
Factor analysis groups items together according to their level of inter-correlation.

- **Exploratory factor analysis** is used to reduce a large number of individual items to a smaller number of relevant concepts, excluding items that do not fit.

- **Confirmatory factor analysis** is used to confirm that items included in an existing scale really do fit together (this is a test of the validity of the scale).

Factor analysis is conceptually similar to thematic analysis in qualitative research – the resulting 'factors' resemble 'common themes' in terms of their interpretation. The difference is that factor analysis is based on numerical scores, not words.

Like qualitative analysis, factor analysis is not an exact science and the researcher must 'choose' the solution that yields factors that make theoretical sense. Unlike qualitative analysis, factor analysis is a complex multivariate statistical test that requires a sample size of at least 100.[2]

---

1 Principal components analysis is a grouping procedure usually used as a preliminary to factor analysis.
2 Tabachnik and Fidell (1989) recommend at least 5 cases (individual respondents) per item. Other authors suggest that 20 cases per item are required to achieve a reliable result.

The first stage of the analysis produces a correlation matrix that identifies the level of association between each of the individual items (for explanation, see Chapter 15). Then a process of extraction groups individual items according to their level of inter-correlation into smaller number of categories or 'factors'.[3] Finally, a process of rotation maximises the separation of these factors to give a solution that is interpretable:

- **Orthogonal rotation** treats each factor as independent from each other factor.

- **Oblique rotation** is used where factors are related and cannot easily be separated.

The results of factor analysis can appear overwhelming because of the large number of procedures and statistics reported. Here, we focus mainly on conceptual interpretation. The ultimate test is whether or not each factor has a coherent set of items that combine to make conceptual sense. Questions to ask include:

1. Do the 'emergent' factors explain a significant percentage of the variance within the data set?

The results give the percentage of the total variance for the data set explained by each individual factor, and by the combined factors. The residual (unexplained) variance includes conceptual and measurement error.

2. Do the items included within each factor share common conceptual meaning (does it make logical sense to group them together)?

This can be looked at in terms of numerical values (factor scores) and common sense.

The SF-36 is a quality of life questionnaire widely used as an outcome measure in medical research. It consists of 36 items grouped into eight scales which are commonly divided into two independent dimensions: a **physical dimension** consisting of physical functioning, physical role function, bodily pain, and general health; and a **mental health dimension** consisting of social functioning, emotional role function, vitality, and mental health.

Hagell et al. (2008) used confirmatory factor analysis to assess if these two dimensions are clinically meaningful for patients with Parkinson's disease, based on a sample of 209 patients. The results are given in Table 6.1.

Example

---

3 Various methods of extraction may be used, the most common of which is referred to as 'maximum likelihood'.

Table 6.1 Table of results for factor analysis (based on data from Hagell et al. 2008)

Items measured	2-factor solution	
	Physical health	Mental health
	Factor scores	
Physical functioning	0.71	0.34
Physical role	0.82	0.34
Bodily pain	0.17	0.74
General health	0.34	0.73
Vitality	0.45	0.76
Social functioning	0.46	0.65
Emotional role	0.81	0.24
Mental health	0.29	0.79
Eigenvalue	4.72	0.76
Variance explained	59%	9.5%
Total variance explained	68.5%	

These 'factor scores' measure the contribution of each item to the factor on a scale from 0 to 1. Minimum score for inclusion in a factor is 0.3

An eigenvalue of at least 1 is usually the minimum for inclusion as a separate factor

Variance explained gives the explanatory power for each factor

Table 6.1 gives the results of factor analysis in a typical format. **Factor scores** are standardised on a scale of 0 to 1 and may be interpreted as follows:

- A score of 0.9 or greater suggests that the item and the factor are virtually indistinguishable. Other items included in the scale are redundant.
- A score of 0.4–0.9 indicates that the item makes an important contribution to the factor.
- Middle range scores of 0.3–0.5 on more than one factor indicate that the factors are not independent of each other.[4]
- A score below 0.3 indicates an item that does not contribute to the factor – these are indicated by shaded cells in Table 6.1.

The 'ideal' solution in factor analysis is one where each item scores reasonably high (preferably 0.4–0.9) on one factor and low (less than 0.3) on each of the others.

An **eigenvalue** is a statistical measure of the significance of each factor. It is usual to eliminate factors with an eigenvalue of less than 1. In Table 6.1, you will see that the eigenvalue for the mental health factor is only 0.76, which might indicate it is not a unique factor.

---

4 In factor analysis, factors that are independent of each other are described as 'orthogonal'.

The **percentage of variance explained** refers to the power of each factor to explain the total variation in the data. It is given as a percentage which is easy to interpret. In Table 6.1, there is a huge imbalance between the two factors: physical health explains 59% of the total variance and mental health only 9.5%. This seems somewhat unlikely, so what is the explanation?

The likely answer is that the first factor extracted uses up all of variance it shares with subsequent factors. So if there is an association between two factors, as is likely between physical and mental health, all of the shared variance (overlap) is attributed to the first factor. The importance of the first factor is thus inflated.

In Table 6.1 the low percentage of variance explained by mental health, combined with an eigenvalue less than 1, suggests that mental and physical health are not clearly distinguishable in patients with Parkinson's disease.

Alternatively, it could mean that items on these scales are ambiguous when applied to this group of patients. For example, our own review of the SF-36 scale items found that the emotional role subscale includes 'task accomplishment', which might explain why it has loaded with items related to physical function in this patient group.

Example

Predictive (criterion) validity

This refers to the power of the measurement scale to predict an objectively verifiable outcome or event. Objective measures might include direct observation of activity or a standardised diagnostic test. An example would be the ability of a depression inventory to predict clinical depression, using clinical interview as the arbiter. Predictive validity may be measured by the percentage of times the correct effect or outcome is predicted.

Concurrent validity

Sometimes it is possible to compare a new measure to an existing validated measure to test how well it measures the same phenomenon. This is often used when a shorter or simpler measure is proposed.

Statistical tests of correlation are used as a measure of success (see Chapter 15 for more information about correlation). Our rule of thumb for interpreting statistical tests of validity and reliability based on correlation (on a scale from 0 to 1) is as follows:

On a scale of 0 (nil) to 1 (perfect):

0.8+	good
0.7–0.79	fairly good
0.6–0.69	just acceptable
<0.6	unacceptable

This is represented visually in Figure 6.1.

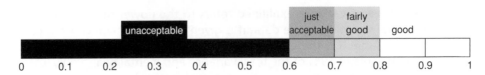

Figure 6.1 Interpretation of 0–1 scores for validity and reliability

Tests of reliability

Reliability refers to the consistency with which the measure performs in practice. There are two types of reliability: **internal consistency,** for which we have Cronbach's alpha (which is also considered a test of construct validity); and **external reliability,** which we can subdivide into test–retest reliability (questionnaire/structure interviews) and inter-rater reliability (direct observation measures).

Internal consistency: Cronbach's alpha (coefficient α)

This measure is widely used to confirm the coherence of a measurement scale or subscale. It is usually used after factor analysis has been used to extract and confirm the presence and structure of independent subscales. It describes how well the selected set of items for each subscale measures a single concept or dimension. Alpha is given on a scale of 0 to 1 which may be interpreted in the same way as concurrent validity (see above).

Example

Ilhan et al. (2008) reported that the Maslach Burnout Inventory has 22 items, each measured using a five-point rating scale. These items are separated into three discrete subscales: Emotional Exhaustion (EE), Depersonalization (DP) and Personal Accomplishment (PA).

The authors do not give Cronbach alpha scores for each of the scales, but a quick internet search using 'Maslach Burnout Inventory + Cronbach' revealed the following alpha values, attributed to the originators Maslach and Jackson: EE = 0.9, DP = 0.79 and PA = 0.71. These all appear fairly good or good using the above criteria.

Note that the value of coefficient alpha increases as the number of items in the scale increases. A score of 0.8 is less impressive if the scale includes 20 items than if it includes only 5 or 6. Similarly, a score of 0.6 might be considered less acceptable if the scale contained more than 10 items.

Test–retest reliability

This reflects the ability of the measure to produce the same result on different occasions when applied under the same conditions. Reliability scores are usually reported on a scale from 0 to 1 and interpreted as for alpha and concurrent validity.

The study by Hagell et al. (2008) included test–retest reliability scores for each of the eight scales measured (Table 6.2). Scores on role scales appear less reliable than the others, possibly because the concepts are less clearly defined. In particular, the reliability of the emotional role scale is only just acceptable at 0.62. It is also worth noting that Hagell et al. report the presence of significant 'floor and ceiling' effects for this scale,[5] which reduced its ability to discriminate between patients with Parkinson's disease.

Table 6.2 Illustration of test–retest reliability scores (based on Hagell et al. 2008)

SF-36 scale	Test–retest reliability
Physical functioning	0.87
Physical role	0.74
Bodily pain	0.86
General health	0.81
Vitality	0.84
Social functioning	0.82
Emotional role	0.62
Mental health	0.84

Inter-rater reliability

This applies to measures based on direct observation. It measures the extent to which two different observers produce similar scores when observing the same events at the same time. There are several ways of measuring inter-rater reliability, including:

- **Correlation**. Where the data are continuous or ordinal, do the scores allocated by the observers closely correlate with each other? A correlation of 0.7 is normally considered the minimum acceptable.

- **Difference**. Does one observer consistently give higher or lower scores than the other? Using a paired test of group difference (Chapter 11) a p value of 0.05 or less ($p \leq 0.05$) indicates that one observer has scored significantly higher than the other, overall.

- **Agreement**. How often do the observers actually agree? Cohen's kappa is a measure of agreement or concordance, based on the number of 'hits' versus

---

5 McHorney and Tarlov (1995) suggest that this applies when more than 15% of the sample achieve either the lowest or highest score in the range.

misses. The following interpretation of kappa is based on Landis and Koch (1977):

<0.20	Poor
0.21–0.40	Fair
0.41–0.60	Moderate
0.61–0.80	Good
0.81–1.00	Very good

The Bland-Altman plot (Altman and Bland 1983) is increasingly recommended to measure inter-rater agreement (and modified for test-retest reliability). Ideally, discrepancy should be zero, though some measurement variation is inevitable. Bias may be judged by the proportion of values that fall either above or below the 95% confidence interval (i.e. mean difference $\pm$ 2 standard deviations).

Summary

Measures of reliability on self-report scales are roughly interpreted as follows:

0.8+	good
0.7–0.79	fairly good
0.6–0.69	just acceptable
<0.6	unacceptable

Further reading

Bland, J.M. and Altman, D.G. (1996) Statistics notes: measurement error and correlation, *British Medical Journal*, 313(7048): 41–2.

At the time of writing (November 2008), a helpful source of free information can be found at http://www.socialresearchmethods.net by following links to knowledge base: measurements.

7 Sampling Data: Probability and Non-probability Samples

KEY QUESTIONS

- Why is the sampling process relevant to the statistical analysis of data?
- How can the sampling process affect the interpretation of the statistical results?
- What clues could indicate sampling bias?
- How should the effects of attrition be addressed?

Introduction

This chapter addresses issues likely to influence the generalisability of research results.

BASIC TERMS
Population or target population refers to everyone or everything sharing a particular characteristic or set of characteristics.
Sample is a group of individuals who have been selected to represent the target population.
Generalisability/generalisation refers to the extent to which the results from the study sample apply to the target population as a whole.
Attrition refers to avoidable and unavoidable losses from the sample following recruitment.

Sampling methods and generalisability

Statistical results are only generalisable to the target population if the sample on which they are based is representative of that population. This means that they must share the same set of characteristics, such as demographic profile (age, gender, social and educational background, etc.), medical profile (disease severity, duration, etc.) and any other factor that could influence or bias the outcome.

Example

The aim of the study by Ilhan et al. (2008) was to determine burnout level and its correlates in nurses (see Chapter 3). In fact it was a study of nurses working in one university hospital in Turkey. This raises a number of questions, such as:

- Is a university hospital comparable to other types of hospital?
- Might nurses in Turkey be qualitatively different from nurses in other parts of the world in terms of their training or attitude to work?
- Might conditions in Turkish hospitals be different from those in other countries?

Factors most likely to affect the generalisability of research findings include:

- inclusion and exclusion criteria;
- the sampling method used;
- self-selection bias and attrition.

Inclusion and exclusion criteria

The inclusion and exclusion criteria determine the target population. Study findings can only be generalised to members of that specific population and not necessarily to any other, so it is important to make a detailed note of these. You will find examples in Chapters 1 and 2.

Sampling method

In this section we briefly discuss a number of sampling methods:

- population sampling;
- random sampling;
- stratified random sampling;
- cluster sampling;
- convenience sampling.

Population sampling

If the target population is small (hundreds rather than thousands) it is wise to recruit all willing participants into the study. If the population is large, it is better to take a sample.

A high response rate from a small(ish) representative sample is better than a poor response rate from a large sample or population (see the discussion by Pincus and Wolfe 2005).

A poor response rate may be an important source of bias and needs to be taken into account when considering the generalisability of the research findings.

Random sampling

Random sampling is the only way of ensuring a truly representative sample. It is often referred to as a 'probability' sample, since all participants share the same probability of being included. Here are two alternative correct methods of random sampling:

- Allocate each potential participant a number. Then select one at a time based on a sequence of numbers taken from a 'table of random numbers'[1] until the required sample size is reached.
- Use computer-generated random sampling – most commonly used these days for large samples.

Random methods assume that all members of the target population are identifiable and contactable.

Pare et al. (2001) wanted to discover the prevalence of constipation in Canada, so they employed a public opinion firm to use a random digital dialling service to invite the participation of at least 1,000 people aged 18 or over in a national survey.

Example

Systematic methods of sampling, such as selecting every third person on the list or every second person through the door do not necessarily produce a representative sample, but are sometimes tempting because random sampling is subject to constraints:

- **Cost**. Only well-funded surveys are likely to be able to achieve a random sample from a large population.
- **Identification**. It is not always possible to identify everyone in the population who meets the inclusion criteria.
- **Access**. Access to many clinical samples is restricted by 'gatekeepers'.

Random sampling operates perfectly in theory, but is difficult to achieve in practice if people fail to respond or participate.

In the Pare et al. study, over 10,000 homes were contacted, of whom 2,000 eligible people were willing to participate. From these, just over 1,000 questionnaires were completed and returned.

Example

---

1 Tables of random numbers are found at the back of most textbooks on statistics.

It is important to check that the researchers did their best to identify if the sample was representative and to examine the data for signs of bias – for example, checking the demographic data to see if the sample characteristics are similar to published data for the target population or other comparable groups.

<table>
<tr><td>Example</td><td>Pare et al. collected demographic data on non-respondents to check there were no systematic differences between respondents and non-respondents.

They also checked against known data to demonstrate that the demographic profile of their sample was proportionate to that of the Canadian population.</td></tr>
</table>

Stratified random sample

This type of random sampling is used if there is known to be an imbalance in subgroups to be compared. From the point of view of statistical tests, the absolute number of each comparison group is important and not the ratio.

Take the example of a study to compare the attributes of male and female nurses. The ratio of males to females on the nursing register is about 1:10. To balance the numbers for comparison, the study included all the male nurses but a 10% random sample of female nurses.

<table>
<tr><td>Example</td><td>Canada is a vast country with two official languages and diverse immigrant and indigenous groups distributed unequally in urban and rural communities across five large regions. Pare et al. needed to ensure that their sample was representative of the population as a whole and also wanted to compare the health of those in the different regions. Therefore the 2,000 people included in the study had been stratified to give 200 participants from each of Canada's ten provinces.</td></tr>
</table>

Cluster sampling

When access to samples is through local 'gatekeepers', such as health professionals, it is acceptable to recruit a random sample from sufficient diverse sites or locations to represent the target population. Whereas stratification starts by identifying the whole target population, cluster sampling starts by identifying only population clusters. It is effective provided the clusters cover all population groups.

Convenience (opportunity) sampling

Many researchers operate on a limited budget and are primarily interested in outcomes in their own location. Therefore it is quite common to find they have used a 'convenience' or 'opportunity' sample.

Convenience sampling refers to a process of approaching and recruiting those readily available to the researcher. It is most commonly used in pilot studies and small-scale surveys. In statistics, it is referred to as a 'non-probability' sample, because it is selective and the results may be susceptible to bias. Therefore it is particularly important to scrutinise the demographic and baseline data for characteristics of the sample or setting that deviate from those encountered in other settings.

Berry et al. (2006) wanted to study public confidence in supplementary nurse prescribing. They conducted a pilot study using a descriptive questionnaire survey. Their sample consisted of 78 people who had never experienced nurse prescribing, recruited at a London station over two consecutive days.

In their discussion, the researchers recognise that a convenience sample of healthy volunteers using public transport at a single location might be biased. Attitudes to nurse prescribing were found to be skewed towards positive attitudes. The researchers acknowledge that the study itself might have induced positive attitudes towards nurses by providing information about nurse prescribing.

Example

Recruitment/response rate

Response rates depend to some extent on the method of approach:

- as low as 10–15% for postal questionnaires with no reminder.
- as high as 50–60% following individual approach.
- A response rate of 100% suggests either strong good will towards the recruiting clinician or some form of coercion! (Yes, we have seen this level of response in a study of mental health patients.)

Reasons for poor response include literacy problems, poor questionnaire design or onerous completion. Long and intrusive questionnaires sent out in the absence of personal contact are particularly likely to produce a poor response.

If the researchers give no indication of the response rate, the reviewer is entitled to ask why. Sometimes the researchers cannot be sure just how many questionnaires were given out, particularly where distribution depends on third parties, but they should make this clear.

Attrition

Attrition refers to loss of data at any stage of the study following recruitment. Since statistics depend on the number (n or N) available for analysis, not the number recruited, this should be clear in the published report.

Atherton et al. (2008) aimed to investigate the effects of attrition in the 1958 British birth cohort study.

- Total in original cohort: 17,638.
- Total in study at age 45: 18,558 (increase due to immigration).
- Unavoidable losses: 1,245 deaths and 1,300 emigrants.
- Eligible total: 16,472.
- Avoidable losses: no contact, 3,004; Non-responders, 3,632.
- Participants: 9,377 (58.6% of eligible participants).

The researchers' analysis showed that socially deprived and ethnic minority groups were under-represented among participants at all ages, and this was increasingly so with age.

We illustrated the relationship between attrition and bias in RCTs in Chapter 1, including a flow diagram identifying attrition at each stage of the study. Things to look out for include:

- Was attrition spread evenly across all intervention or population groups?
- If not, is an explanation offered for the disparity and is there any likely source of systematic bias?

Missing data

Self-report questionnaires used in surveys or RCTs are susceptible to the failure of participants to complete all parts of all questions, leading to missing data. Note that the number (n) of respondents or subjects included in each statistical analysis is the one that counts, *not* the number of questionnaires returned. Missing data can leave the analysis with insufficient data to detect a significant result, if there is one to be found (Type II error).

For each statistical analysis, look carefully at the value of n (number of cases) or df (degrees of freedom[2]) to see if this is considerably less than the original sample size. If there is a discrepancy, is this accounted for?

Intention-to-treat analysis

Intention-to-treat analysis is used in RCTs to compensate for systematic bias caused by attrition (see the example in Chapter 1). It involves substituting a score in place of missing data at follow-up. This usually assumes no benefit – i.e.

---

2 Degrees of freedom (df) is closely related to the number of cases included in the analysis, usually equal to $n - 1$. This small correction is designed to avoid over-estimating the strength of a relationship in small samples but is not relevant in samples of over 100.

drop-outs are allocated the same score at post-test as they recorded at baseline. Other methods include substituting an average group score. It should be clear what substitutions were made, and these should be sure to address potential sources of bias in study outcome.

Summary

- Only a large random sample is truly representative of the target population.
- Generalisation of the results is restricted by sampling bias, inclusion and exclusion criteria, response rate and attrition.
- Poor response and attrition are important source bias.

8 Sample Size: Criteria for Judging Adequacy

KEY QUESTIONS

- How do I judge if the sample size is large enough?
- What factors influence sample size?
- What specific sampling issues apply to RCTs and surveys?

Introduction

The question all reviewers want answered is: 'was the sample size large enough?' That begs the question: 'large enough for what?' The answer is surprisingly complex.

The minimum sample size is one that will detect a statistically significant result if there is one to be found. Sample size calculation involves a mathematical formula that takes account of the following:

- the statistical tests planned;
- level of statistical power (accuracy) required;
- level of probability (value of α) set as significant;
- strength and direction of the principal hypotheses (see Chapter 9);
- size of the outcome or effect to be detected;
- size of subgroups to be compared;
- response rate and attrition.

These details should be found in the Method section of the research paper under the heading of 'Data analysis' or similar. In this chapter, we give a brief overview of key issues related to each aspect, followed by specific issues related to RCTs and surveys.

BASIC TERMS

Parametric refers to the normal distribution curve.

Nonparametric refers to data and statistical tests that do not conform to, or depend on, the normal distribution curve.

Planned statistical tests

Each test depends on:

- the nature of the research question or hypothesis;
- the type and distribution of the dependent (outcome) variable;
- the complexity of the analysis.

Table 8.1 contains a rough guide to sample sizes, based on these factors. These are the *minimum* sample sizes required, assuming at least a moderate effect to be detected, and fairly even distribution of the data.

Table 8.1 Rough guide to minimum sample sizes

Purpose	Continuous data	Categorical data
Compare groups	t test, ANOVA: $n \geq 30$ in each group (see Redmond and Keenan 2002)[a]	Contingency analysis (chi-square): $n > 50$ (2 groups, 2 categories) $n > 60$ (2 groups, 3 categories)
Correlate 2 variables	Pearson correlation (r): $n \geq 30$	
Multivariate analysis	Multiple regression, factor analysis: $n \geq 100$ if there are up to 5 independent (predictor) variables; add 20 for each additional independent variable	Logistic regression: $n > 400$

[a] These are sometimes referred to as 'univariate' because there is one dependent variable.

Additional notes on categorical (nominal) data

The requirements for contingency analysis of categorical data are unique and specific:

- For a 2 × 2 table (two groups, two categories of response), a minimum 'expected' frequency of 10 in each cell (category of response) is recommended (see Chapter 11). This gives a minimum sample size requirement of 40, assuming that there are equal numbers in each group and an even balance of response. A minimum sample size of 50 is recommended to compensate for modest imbalances in the expected distribution.
- For a larger table (more groups or categories of response), at least 80% of cells must contain a minimum 'expected' frequency of 5 for the analysis to be valid (expected frequencies are those that are found if there is no observed effect; see Chapter 11 for more details). Allowing for imbalances in distribution, this necessitates a much larger sample size.

Researchers often run into problems because they fail to anticipate unequal or uneven distributions. This is a particular problem where comparisons between subgroups are determined after the data has already been collected.

The research question in Jebb et al. (2003) was: 'is there a sex difference in the prevalence of overweight and obesity at different ages?' The researchers collected categorised data from a national random sample of children. In calculating their sample size, they needed to ensure that it would include sufficient numbers of obese boys and girls in each age group for the purpose of comparison. The final sample size was 1,667 children. But you can see from Table 8.2 that the numbers in some obese categories were very small.

Table 8.2 Contingency table showing breakdown of actual and expected numbers in each 'cell' (from Jebb et al. 2003)

Prevalence of obesity and overweight in a national random sample of 859 boys and 808 girls by age					
	Actual *n* (expected *n*) Boys		Actual *n* (expected *n*) Girls		
Age group	Overweight	Obese	Overweight	Obese	TOTALS
4–6	27	4 (5.5)	32	6 (7.4)	69
7–8	13	1 (2.9)	19	4 (4)	37
9–11	24	9 (6)	37	6 (8.2)	76
12–14	30	4 (4.8)	17	10 (6.6)	61
15–17	32	7 (5.7)	25	8 (7.8)	72
TOTALS	126	25	130	34	315

Total obese boys

Expected frequencies in brackets

Total children age 7–8

Total overweight and obese children

There are two independent (predictor) variables (sex and age) and one dependent (effect) variable (obesity):

- age has five categories;
- sex has two categories;
- weight has two categories.

The total number of cells to be filled is 5 (age) × 2 (sex) × 2 (weight) = 20.

To ensure a minimum of 5 expected observations in 80% of these cells would require a sample size of 80% × (20 × 5) = 80. But this would make no allowance at all for any imbalance in the ratios for gender, age and weight.

In fact, these researchers carefully based their sample size calculation on known data for the proportions of obese boys and girls in the population. This ensured that they were able to meet the sample size requirement for these comparisons.

Statistical power

Statistical power refers to the level of accuracy or precision required of the statistical analysis. No statistical test is 100% accurate. Normally 80% power is considered to be sufficient, but in clinical trials that carry a high risk of unwanted side-effects the power is normally raised to 90%. This raises the threshold for significant benefit where there is a risk of adverse events. An increase in power requires a larger sample size to detect a statistically significant difference (assuming there is one) and is only feasible in the context of a large and well-funded clinical trial.

Significance level, α

It is usually accepted that a significance level set at $\alpha = 0.05$ (i.e. $p \leq 0.05$) is adequate to test a hypothesis (see Chapter 9). This represents a likelihood of 5% or less that there is *no* difference between groups or association between variables (remember, statistical tests test the null hypothesis). In other words, there is a 95% likelihood that the results support researcher's hypothesis – the result is statistically significant.

A more stringent test of significance set, for example, at $\alpha = 0.01$, would require a larger sample size. Table 8.3 gives an extract from the statistical table for the Pearson correlation coefficient, r, assuming that $r = 0.3$ (a weak to moderate effect). It illustrates the increase in sample size required to detect different levels of statistical significance, given the same level of correlation in the data.

Table 8.3 Extract from statistical table for Pearson correlation coefficient, $r = 0.3$ (moderate)

n	Significance (one-tailed), $r = 0.3$
20	$p > 0.05$, not significant (ns)
30	$p = 0.05$
40	$p = 0.02$
50	$p = 0.01$
80	$p = 0.005$
100	$p = 0.001$

Situations where the significance level needs to be set at a more stringent level (e.g. $\alpha = 0.01$, $p \leq 0.01$) include:

- In surveys where a lot of comparisons or correlations are planned. For example, if 20 comparisons are made, at least one false positive result may be expected if the significance level is set at $\alpha = 0.05$ (1 in 20). The significance level required to avoid Type I error (a false significant result) may be determined using the Bonferroni correction (see Chapter 9).
- In clinical trials where risks associated with overestimation of treatment efficacy are high.

The strength and direction of the hypothesis to be tested

If the researchers present an evidence-based rationale for predicting a positive or negative difference between groups or relationship between variables, a directional (one-tailed) test of probability is justified. Otherwise a non-directional (two-tailed) test of probability must be applied (see Chapter 9).

A two-tailed test of probability requires a much larger sample size to achieve a statistically significant result. This is illustrated in Table 8.4, based on data from statistical tables for the Pearson correlation coefficient r.

Table 8.4 Comparison of sample sizes required to achieve a statistically significant result for different values of r using a one-tailed and a two-tailed test of probability

Test result: value of r	Approx. sample size required to achieve a statistically significant result for one-tailed test ($p \leq 0.05$)	Approx. sample size required to achieve a statistically significant result for two-tailed test ($p \leq 0.05$)
0.2	65	100
0.3	30	42
0.4	18	23

The researchers should indicate the test of probability used when calculating the sample size for their study. If they do not, the reviewer should check that the correct test was applied. This can be achieved using statistical tables (see Part 3 for further guidance).

The size of effect

By 'effect' we mean a clinically important or meaningful change or difference. The **effect size** is a standardised measure of difference or sensitivity to change. For example, when comparing a measurable outcome between two groups, as in a clinical trial, the effect size is calculated as:

$$\text{Effect size} = \frac{\text{mean of experimental group} - \text{mean of control group}}{\text{standard deviation}}.$$

In this equation,[1] the difference between the group means is the measure of treatment effect considered to be clinically important (see the example in Chapter 1).

- The larger the treatment effect predicted, the larger the effect size and the smaller the sample size required to detect it.
- The larger the standard deviation for the measurement used, the smaller the effect size and the larger the sample size required to detect an effect.

Effect size is a standardised value which applies regardless of the measurement scale used. The following interpretation of effect size (from Cohen 1988) is generally accepted as a rough approximation:

---

1 You may recognise it as the formula used to calculate the value of t in the t test (see Chapter 10).

≥ 0.8 is large.

0.5–0.8 is moderate (0.5 is usually the minimum effect size considered acceptable in an RCT).

0.2–0.5 is small.

Anything smaller than 0.1 is trivial.

In an RCT, effect size can be thought of in terms of the extent of overlap between the same set of measurements taken from two treatment groups. The greater the overlap, the smaller the effect size and the smaller the difference between the two groups:

- An effect size of 0 indicates total (100%) overlap. There is absolutely no difference between the two groups.
- An effect size of 0.8 indicates an overlap of approximately 53%.
- An effect size of 1.7 indicates an overlap of approximately 25%.

To give effect size more general meaning, Coe (2000) explains that in the UK, the distribution of GCSE grades in maths and English are such that an improvement of one GCSE grade represents an effect size of between 0.5 and 0.7.

The smaller the predicted effect size, the larger the sample size required to detect a difference or relationship in the data. Researchers often base their sample size calculation on an estimated effect size of 0.5 for the primary outcome measure. To ensure that this is realistic, it must be supported by published evidence or pilot study data.

An effect size based on published data assumes that the research sample is taken from a similar target population, likely to respond in the same way.

If an RCT uses an untested dependent measure or one tested using a different population, it is necessary to conduct a phase 2 clinical trial. This should include at least 100 participants in order to estimate the size of treatment effect and standard deviation for the main outcome measure, since these are the key components of effect size.[2]

Richards et al. (2008) conducted a randomised phase 2 study to calculate the effect size for collaborative care for depression, in preparation for a full-scale clinical trial. They used one primary outcome measure of depression, the Patient Health Questionnaire (PHQ9) and some general quality of life measures. For this pilot study, they recruited 114 patients, distributed between one intervention group, one randomised control group and one cluster control group.

Based on treatment differences between the intervention group and the cluster control group, and standard deviations, the effect size was calculated as 0.63 (moderate). This was used as a basis for their sample size calculation.

Example

2 For more information about phase 1, 2 and 3 trials, see http://www.cancerhelp.org.uk/help/default.asp?page=73

Effect sizes can be calculated for other types of statistical analysis, such as correlation, regression and chi-square. These are based on formulæ specific to those tests and different standards for judging effect size. These are beyond the scope of this book but can be found on internet sites, such as www.researchconsultation.com (at the time of writing).

The most important thing is to note if the researchers give the criteria they used to calculate their sample size.

Response rate and attrition

It is important to note if the researchers made adequate allowance at the planning stage for the likely response rate and attrition. Some sources recommend an allowance of 15% for attrition following recruitment into an intervention study with follow-up (we addressed these issues in some detail in Chapter 7).

Example

Hagen et al. (2003) conducted a descriptive survey to identify the proportion of children attending a hospital rheumatology clinic who used complementary or alternative medicine (CAM).

Based on pilot data, Hagen et al. estimated CAM use at 65%. Based on this, they estimated an available sample size of 180 out of the total population of 277 children attended the clinic.

Hagen et al. anticipated a response rate from random mailing of 80%, giving a sample size requirement of 144. This proved to be over-optimistic. The actual response rate was 46.4%, compared to 100% for the patients who were approached in person.

Sample size calculation for an RCT (power calculation)

This needs to answer the following question: *what is the minimum sample size required to be reasonably certain of detecting a significant difference between the intervention and the control group(s), assuming there is a difference to be found?*

In answer, the researcher should state:

- the statistical power required (80% or 90%);
- the effect size (or the clinically important effect and standard deviation for the main measures);
- the significance level set (level of α);
- the test of probability applied (usually two-tailed in an RCT);
- allowance for attrition.

Graff et al. (2006) described an RCT designed to compare the outcomes of an occupational therapy intervention for dementia patients with usual care. The researchers gave details of the criteria used to determine their sample size (see Table 8.5).

Example

Table 8.5 Example of sample size criteria (from Graff et al. 2006)

Outcome measure used	Range of values	Clinical effect required
Process skill	−3 to +4	0.5 scale points
Activity performance	0 to 40	20% improvement
Sense of competence	27 to 435	5 points

The researchers specify a statistical power of 80%, a significance level of 0.05 and one-tailed probability tests (though two-tailed tests were used in actual analyses). Standard deviations and effect sizes are not given, but appear to be known from earlier research carried out by the research team.

The researchers state that their power calculation determined that at least 100 full sets of pre- and post-test responses were needed to achieve all of the desired outcomes.

You will find a further example in Chapter 1.

Sample sizes for descriptive surveys

In a purely descriptive survey, the aim is to generalize information from the sample to the target population (see Chapter 2). Table 8.6 summarises advice by Bartlett et al. (2001) on minimum sample sizes.[3]

Table 8.6 shows that the sample size is not directly proportional to the population size. Note that these sample sizes assume a non-directional, two-tailed

Table 8.6 Guidelines on minimum sample sizes for descriptive survey (Bartlett et al. 2001)

Population size	Sample size (*n*) for two-tailed test, $p \leq 0.05$	
	Continuous data	Categorical data
100	55	80
300	85	169
500	96	218
1000	106	278
10,000	119	370

3 Note that other sources give different advice.

significance level set at $\alpha = 0.05$. Note also that the sample size, n, refers to the number of *complete* sets of data available for analysis.

Sample size calculations for analytic surveys

Epidemiological and health survey data is usually subjected to a series of simple tests, including correlation, followed by sophisticated statistical analysis, such as multiple or logistic regression. For sample size requirements, we refer back to Table 8.1. It is usual to base the sample size calculation on the most complex multivariate tests used in the study. You will find an example based on multiple regression in Chapter 2.

Sample size calculation for logistic regression is particularly complex because it depends on the odds ratio considered necessary to express a clinically important effect (see Chapter 16), and the expected distribution for each predictor variable.

Example

Broll et al. (2002) present a detailed account of their sample size calculation for a German veterinary study of risk factors for toxoplasmosis in pregnant women. The dependent (outcome) variable in logistic regression analysis was the presence or absence of toxoplasmosis. The two predictor variables were 'consumption of raw meat' and 'cat ownership'. The following predictors were based on published data from Germany and Switzerland:

- cat ownership 14%;
- raw meat consumption 38% (data from 1973);
- odds ratio of 2 should be detectable;
- $p \leq 0.05$.

Assuming that cat ownership was the risk factor of primary interest, the researchers estimated their required sample size to be at least 742.

The above example is actually a very simple one. There is one dichotomous outcome variable (toxoplasmosis present or absent) and two dichotomous predictors. The reason for the large sample size is that the estimated proportion of cat owners is quite small.

Any imbalance in the distribution of an independent variable increases the sample size requirement. Therefore it is extremely important that the researchers demonstrate the steps taken to predict the likely distribution when estimating their required sample size.

Summary

Researchers should clearly state the criteria used to predict the minimum sample size requirement for their data analysis, including:

- the significance level and direction of the hypothesis;
- the type of data and planned statistical tests;
- the size of groups for comparison;
- the effect size, or clinically important effect and standard deviation, for each primary outcome measure;
- predicted attrition.

Further reading

See Bandolier (2008) on the classification of effect size. It is also worth looking at some of the academic websites from well-established universities in the UK or USA.

Commercial sites also offer useful basic information. At the time of writing, www.researchconsultation.com gives useful advice to students on sample size calculation.

For those who wish to further their mathematical understanding, the journal *Statistics in Medicine* provides articles on all aspects of statistical analysis.

9 Testing Hypotheses:
What Does *p* Actually Mean?

KEY QUESTIONS

- What is a hypothesis and how do statistics test it?
- What is meant by the 'null hypothesis' and why is it important?
- What is meant by Type I and Type II (types one and two) error?
- What does *p* mean?
- What is meant by 'significance level'?
- What is the difference between a directional (one-tailed) test and a non-directional (two-tailed) test of probability and why is this important?
- What is the difference between statistical significance and clinical importance?
- What is meant by a confidence interval?

Introduction

Each statistical test consists of a unique mathematical algorithm (calculation) which is designed to test a hypothesis about a difference between groups or a relationship between variables. These tests provide an answer in terms of the probability or likelihood that there is *no* difference between groups or *no* relationship between variables. In other words, they test the 'null hypothesis'.

In order to determine statistical significance, the research community decides at which point the result of the statistical analysis ceases to uphold the null hypothesis. It is generally agreed that this threshold occurs when the probability that there is no difference or association in the data is 5% (1:20) or less. This 'significance level' is indicated by $\alpha = 0.05$ ($p \leq 0.05$).

Figure 9.1 illustrates key stages in the research process from the development of the hypothesis to the decision about whether to accept or reject the null hypothesis (and by implication to reject or accept the researcher's hypothesis).[1]

In this chapter, we explain significance testing and explore factors that need to be taken into account when judging whether or not a research result is statistically significant.

---

1 Strictly speaking, a statistician would *fail to reject* the null hypothesis, rather than accept it.

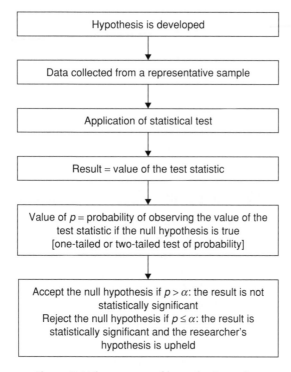

Figure 9.1 The process of hypothesis testing

BASIC TERMS
Hypothesis predicts a difference between two or more groups or a relationship
   between two or more variables.
Null hypothesis states that there will be *no* difference between the groups, or
   no relationship between the variables.
Type I error occurs when the researcher's hypothesis is held to be true when it
   is actually not true.
Type II error occurs when the researcher's hypothesis is rejected when it is
   actually true.
p **(probability)** is given as a value, in decimals, between 0 and 1.
α **(alpha)** is the significance level set for the study.

What is a hypothesis?

A hypothesis is a prediction based on sound theory, previous research evidence,
or informed speculation. It is presented in the form of a statement of the likely
outcome. There are two types of hypothesis that are tested using statistical tests:

- The prediction of a difference between two or more groups, answered using
  a test of group difference (see Chapters 11 and 12).

- The prediction of an association between two or more variables, answered
  using a test of correlation or regression (see Chapter 15).

The researcher's hypothesis takes one of two distinct forms:

- A directional prediction that there will be a difference or relationship in the data, and this will be in one direction only (known as one-tailed).
- A non-directional prediction that there may be a difference or relationship, but the existence or direction of the relationship is not entirely certain (known as two-tailed).

These forms of hypothesis determine the test of probability applied to the statistical result, and hence their statistical significance. The researchers state a hypothesis in one of these forms, but statistical tests all test the null hypothesis.

What is the null hypothesis and why is it important?

The null hypothesis states that there will be *no* difference between groups, or *no* relationship between the selected variables. It is an important concept in statistics because all statistical tests start from the premise that the null hypothesis is true and remains so unless or until statistical testing proves otherwise. The null hypothesis is an implicit assumption that underpins statistical tests – researchers do not need to state it.

What does *p* mean?

The value of *p* gives the level of probability that the null hypothesis is true and there is *no* difference between groups or *no* association between variables. The smaller the value of *p*, the smaller the likelihood that the null hypothesis is true and the greater the likelihood that the researcher's hypothesis is true. Thus the smaller the value of *p* (e.g. more zeros after the decimal point), the greater the statistical significance of the research results.

Table 9.1 interprets a range of *p* values for those not familiar with them.

Table 9.1 Examples of *p* values and their interpretation

$p \leq 0.05$	This test result is likely to be observed less than five times out of every hundred occasions (5:100 or 1:20) if there really is no difference or association. This is usually considered sufficiently unlikely as to be termed 'statistically significant'.
$p < 0.01$	This result is likely to occur less than once out of every hundred times (1:100). This is considered very unlikely and hence very significant.
$p \leq 0.001$	This result is likely to occur once in a thousand times (1:1000) or less. This is considered to be highly unlikely and hence highly significant.
$p > 0.05$	The result is likely to occur more than five times out of every hundred (5:100 or 1:20). This is deemed to be within the range of normal occurrence and is not 'statistically significant'. The result is often recorded as 'ns' (not significant).
$p = 0.1$	This result is likely to occur 10% of the time. It is not statistically significant.
$p = 0.5$	This result is likely to occur 50% of the time. It is not statistically significant.
$p = 0.79$	This result is likely to occur 79% of the time. It is not statistically significant.

Probability is always given in decimals on a scale of 0 to 1, though it equates to a percentage or ratio:

$p = 0.05$ is the same as 5% or 5:100 or 1:20;

$p = 0.01$ is the same as 1% or 1:100

What is meant by 'significance level'?

The scientific community decides the point at which the result of a statistical test ceases to uphold the null hypothesis. It is generally agreed that the minimum threshold occurs when the likelihood that there is *no* effect is 5% (1:20) or less. This 'significance level' is indicated by $\alpha = 0.05$ ($p \leq 0.05$).

The significance level is often referred to as the **level of alpha**.[2] The default significance level is set at $\alpha = 0.05$. This indicates a 5% probability or less that the results showed no difference or association. This gives a likelihood of 95% or more that a real difference or association has been observed.

The cut-off point for statistical significance at $\alpha = 0.05$ ($p \leq 0.05$) is absolute. Any result given as a probability greater than 0.05 is not statistically significant. As the threshold for statistical significance is raised, the value of α is decreased. For example, if α is set at 0.01, the value of p in the results must be ≤ 0.01 to achieve significance.

Claesson et al. (2007) conducted an intervention study to promote weight control in obese women during pregnancy. Preliminary analysis gave results for tests of group difference between the intervention and the control group at baseline.

Which, if any, of the p values in Table 9.2 would you classify as statistically significant if $\alpha = 0.05$?

Example

Table 9.2 Examples of p values (from Claesson et al. 2007)

	Value of p
Age	0.307
Marital status	0.853
Smoking	0.695
BMI	0.948
Socio-economic status (SES)	0.044
Occupation	0.160

There is only one significant value of p (i.e. $p < 0.05$) in this list: a significant difference between groups is reported for SES ($p = 0.044$).

---

2 Not to be confused with 'coefficient alpha' in Chapter 4.

Why do some researchers set a different significance level?

The significance level may need to be changed in order to reduce the likelihood of Type I error (obtaining a false significant result). A smaller value of p is set as significant where:

- the scientific outcome needs to be very safe or certain, as in some drug trials where there is a risk of side-effects;
- multiple comparisons are made, since more test results provide more opportunities for achieving a false positive outcome.

Example

A researcher reports on the evaluation of an intervention to improve pain, mobility and quality of life in people with a chronic health problem. Outcome measures included:

4 scales of pain measurement;

3 scales of mobility;

2 scales of disability;

2 measures of depression;

2 measures of anxiety;

2 measures of anger/hostility;

5 scales of quality of life.

There are thus 20 outcome variables. Each is tested individually to see if it distinguishes between the intervention and control group. A significance level of $\alpha = 0.05$ was set. Consider the following results:

- On 10 of the outcome measures, patients in the intervention group showed no improvement compared to the control group for 10 ($p > 0.05$, ns).
- On the remaining outcome measures, the p value is given as ≤ 0.05.

How would you interpret these results?

In this case, the researchers might be criticised for attempting to test too many outcome variables in a single piece of research. Given that there were 20 separate statistical tests, at least one false significant result (Type I error) is likely to occur if the significance level is set at 0.05 (1:20). But which one?

To help protect against Type I error where multiple statistical tests are used, the value of p needs to be reduced. The Bonferroni correction is the most common way of identifying the appropriate level of reduction.

Bonferroni correction

The Bonferroni correction is commonly used to change the level of alpha where a series of statistical tests are carried out on the same set of data.

The Bonferroni correction uses the formula $\alpha \div n$, where α is the significance level that normally would be set (usually $\alpha = 0.05$) and n represents the number of statistical tests planned.

In the previous example, 20 comparisons were made. Using the Bonferroni correction, the adjustment would be $0.05 \div 20$, giving $\alpha = 0.0025$. This would mean that none of the researcher's findings was statistically significant.

The Bonferroni correction remains controversial with researchers who argue it is too stringent and increases the incidence of Type II error (failure to find a significant result where there really is one). Where used, the Bonferroni correction should be taken into account by researchers when calculating their sample size at the planning stage (the smaller the value of α, the larger the sample size needed to detect a statistically significant result, if there is one).

One-tailed (directional) versus two-tailed (non-directional) tests of probability

From a statistical perspective a hypothesis can take two forms:

1. A confident and precise prediction that there will be a difference between groups or a relationship between variables and that this will occur in one direction only. This is referred to as a directional, one-tailed or one-sided hypothesis. For example:

   • The intervention group will show a greater reduction in weight gain during pregnancy than the control group.
   • Higher saturated fat intake will be associated with an increase in blood cholesterol.

2. A prediction that there may be a difference or association, but this is not entirely certain and/or it is not clear in what direction this relationship will be. This is referred to as a non-directional, two-tailed or two-sided hypothesis. For example:

   • Men and women will differ in their attitudes towards health education material.
   • Self-reported well-being may be associated with age.

Directional testing and critical values

Why is a directional test of probability referred to as one-tailed? Why is a non-directional test of probability referred to as two-tailed?

The range of values for each test statistic conforms to the normal distribution, with a standard deviation that depends on the sample size.

The 'tails' refer to the extreme ends or tails of the distribution of test statistic values, as represented in Figure 9.2. The 'critical values' are the cut-off points for different levels of probability.

In Figure 9.2, the shaded areas indicate the 95% of the area under the normal distribution represented by the null hypothesis. Assuming the significance level is $\alpha = 0.05$:

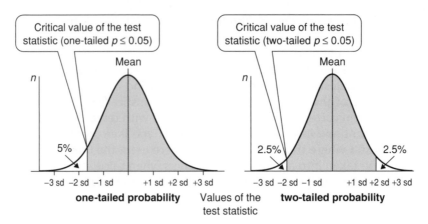

Figure 9.2 Comparison of one-tailed (directional) and two-tailed (non-directional) tests of probability

- In the one-tailed test of probability, all 5% of test results labelled 'significant' are loaded at one end of the distribution.
- In the two-tailed test of probability, the 5% of significant test results are loaded equally at each end of the distribution.

A smaller critical value is required to achieve statistical significance if a one-tailed test of probability is applied, making it more likely that the test result will be defined as statistically significant.

In effect, one-tailed $p \leq 0.05$ is equivalent to two-tailed $p \leq 0.025$. A two-tailed test reduces the likelihood of overestimating the significance of an outcome that could not be predicted with reasonable certainty. The researcher is only justified in applying a one-tailed test of probability if they are able to offer persuasive justification for their hypothesis in their introduction.

The values of p for each statistical test are programmed into statistical computer packages and printed out automatically – but the onus is on researchers to ensure that the correct test of probability (one-tailed or two-tailed) has been applied. They should report in their Method section which test of probability was applied.

Example

Mangunkusumo et al. (2007) presented a complex intervention study designed to test whether the acceptance of interactive health promotion material by teenagers could be enhanced using the internet, compared to traditional paper and pencil (P&P) methods. The Introduction makes it clear that although the internet was a more efficient method of delivery, there was no evidence to support one approach over the other in terms of outcomes.

In accordance with this, the researchers state in their section on data analysis that differences between the internet and P&P groups were tested using two-tailed tests with an alpha of 0.05.

Occasionally, the researchers fail to state whether a one-tailed or a two-tailed test was applied. If there is doubt, it is possible to check the value of the test statistic against the value of p using a set of statistical tables. These are found at the back of standard textbooks on statistics, or on academic or commercial internet sites. We have included extracts in Part 4 as a rough guide.

Table 9.3 illustrates how to use statistical tables, based on the independent t test, used to compare two groups (see Chapter 11).

Table 9.3 Interpretation of statistical table for the t test (critical values of t are given in the shaded cells)

Degrees of freedom = total number of observations − 2

Values of t in this column are significant if one-tailed p is applied ($p = 0.05$) but not if two-tailed p is applied ($p = 0.1$)

	Directional (one-tailed) p				
	0.05	0.025	0.01	0.005	0.0005
	Non-directional (two-tailed) p				
df $(n − 2)$[a]	0.1	0.05	0.02	0.01	0.001
20	1.7	2.1	2.5	2.8	3.9
30	1.7	2.0	2.5	2.8	3.6
60	1.7	2.0	2.4	2.7	3.5
120+	1.6	2.0	2.3	2.6	3.3

Each critical value of t represents the minimum value required to achieve statistical significance at the level indicated at the top of the column.
  In this column, the value of t must be at least 2.0 to achieve one-tailed $p = 0.025$ or two-tailed $p = 0.05$ if n is greater than 30.

Critical values of t vary with sample size and with level of probability

[a] The t test is based on degrees of freedom rather than sample size in order to reduce the chances of overestimating significance when the sample size is small.

Table 9.3 illustrates that if the researcher gives the result as $t = 2.8$ with df $= 30$ ($n = 32$), the above table will confirm the result as $p \leq 0.005$ (one-tailed) or $p \leq 0.01$ (two-tailed).

Example

Note the following:

- As the values of t increase, the values of p decrease, thus increasing the statistical significance of the test result.
- The values of t are sensitive to sample size. The same value of t is more likely to achieve significance as the sample size increases.
- A one-tailed test of probability is more likely to give a statistically significant result than a two-tailed test of probability.

Similar observations apply to all other statistical tests. We give more details about 'critical values' in Chapter 10.

Does it really matter if the researcher uses a one-tailed or two-tailed test of probability?

Yes, it can make a big difference! The same value of the test statistic gives a different level of probability, depending on whether a directional (one-tailed) or non-directional (two-tailed) test of probability is applied. In some cases, this can make the difference between a significant and a non-significant outcome. Table 9.4 compares values of t using one-tailed and two-tailed tests.

Table 9.4 Extract from a statistical table for the t test, comparing values of t that achieve significance using one-tailed and two-tailed tests of probability

df ($n - 2$)	Critical value of t (one-tailed, $p = 0.05$)	Critical value of t (two-tailed, $p = 0.05$)
20	1.73	2.09
60	1.67	2.00
120	1.66	1.98

Type I error and Type II error (Types one and two error)

These types of statistical error are illustrated in Table 9.5.

Table 9.5 Type I versus Type II error

	Researcher's hypothesis is TRUE	Researcher's hypothesis is FALSE
Result IS statistically significant	Correct decision	False positive outcome TYPE I ERROR
Result IS NOT statistically significant	False negative outcome TYPE II ERROR	Correct decision

Type I error refers to a false positive result. It occurs when a statistically significant outcome is reported when none actually exists. Reasons for this include:

- the failure to reduce the significance level from $\alpha = 0.05$ to, say $\alpha = 0.01$, when using multiple statistical tests (see Bonferroni correction);
- the incorrect use of a directional (one-tailed) test of probability when a non-directional (two-tailed) test of probability should have been used.

Type II error refers to a false negative result. It occurs when a real difference or association is found to be non-significant. Reasons for this include:

- inadequate sample size;
- the use of insensitive or unreliable measurements.

These reasons are all avoidable if researchers design and implement their study with due care. They are also good reasons why a reviewer should never take research results at face value.

What is the difference between statistical significance and clinical importance?

A result can only be judged to be clinically important if it is statistically significant. But a statistically significant result obtained from a very large sample may be too small to be considered clinically important or relevant.

How is clinical relevance established?

Clinical importance or relevance in a clinical trial refers to a level of improvement judged to be of clinical benefit. It determines 'effect size' which in turn influences sample size.

Recognised ways of establishing a clinically important improvement include:

- Existing epidemiological or other research-based evidence to demonstrate the change necessary to bring about health improvement.
- Professional judgement about the improvement needed to reduce care needs.
- Patient involvement to establish the improvement needed for a positive effect on their quality of life.

What is meant by 'approaching significance'?

The significance level should be determined before the study commences and is absolute. The results either achieve it or they do not. Researchers sometimes argue that a result might have been significant had the sample size been larger. If that is the case, they should have calculated their sample size to ensure it was adequate to detect a significant result. There is no way of knowing, after the event, if the result would have achieved significance had the sample size been larger.

What is meant by a confidence interval?

A confidence interval (CI) gives the range of values that predict the true value for the target population with the degree of certainty specified (e.g. 95% or

99%). The relationship between confidence interval and significance level is illustrated by the equation

$$CI = (1 - \alpha) \times 100\%$$

where α is the level of probability set as the significance level. CI and α are complementary. It just happens that α is given as a decimal and the confidence interval is given as a percentage.

- A 95% confidence interval is given where the significance level is set at $\alpha = 0.05$ ($p \leq 0.05$).
- A 99% confidence interval is given where the significance level is set at $\alpha = 0.01$ ($p \leq 0.01$).

The confidence interval provides an increasingly accepted way of conveying clinically relevant research findings. No test result is precise and the range of values predicted with reasonable certainty is clinically more meaningful.

- If both values of the CI are on the same side of zero, the result is statistically significant.
- If zero lies between the two values (i.e. if one value is positive and the other negative), the result is not statistically significant.

Summary

- The value of p reflects the probability that the null hypothesis is true (there are no differences between groups and/or no associations between variables.
- The significance level (level of alpha) is the value of p judged likely to exclude false positive findings (Type I error).
- A one-tailed test of probability must only be used if there is sufficient evidence to support a directional hypothesis.
- The significance level, α, must minimise Type I error.
- The confidence interval (CI) used in the results is complementary to the significance level used.

Further reading

Redmond, A.C. and Keenan, A.-M. (2002) Understanding statistics: putting p-values into perspective. *Journal of the American Podiatric Medical Association*, 92: 297–305.

PART 3
STATISTICAL TESTS

This section explains statistical tests in common use. To make sense of these, you will need the following knowledge base:

- types of data (see Chapter 3);
- distribution of data (see Chapters 4 and 5);
- hypothesis testing (see Chapter 9).

10 Introduction to Inferential Statistics

KEY QUESTIONS

- What is meant by the term 'inferential statistics'?
- What are the main types of test used and what is their purpose?
- What determines the appropriate choice of test?
- What factors influence the statistical results?
- How are statistical results normally presented?

Introduction

The statistical tests described in this part of the book are called 'inferential' because the results generate inferences, in the form of probability, that are generalisable to the population from which the study sample is drawn. Note that all of these tests are based on the assumption that the research sample is representative of the target population. This requires a random or 'probability' sample (see Chapter 7).

ESSENTIAL TERMINOLOGY

Null hypothesis. Statistical tests test the null hypothesis which predicts there will be *no* effect.

p denotes the probability that the null hypothesis is true.

df = degrees of freedom. Closely related to sample or category size, but with small adjustment to reduce overestimating statistical significance.

Parametric refers to data that conform to the normal distribution and tests that depend on the normal distribution.

Nonparametric refers to data and tests that do not fulfil the assumption of normal distribution.

What are the main types of test and what is their purpose?

Each statistical test is designed to answer a specific research question or test a specific type of hypothesis:

- Tests of group difference or comparison look for differences between the same set of measurements taken from one or more groups of individuals.

- Tests of association (correlation and regression) test for a relationship between two or more sets of measurements taken from the same group of (or matched) individuals.

Some tests, such as ANOVA, combine these features.

What determines which test should be used?

Key criteria for judging the appropriate use of a statistical test include:

- The nature of the hypothesis tested – is it to compare groups or identify associations between variables?
- The number of groups or variables included in the analysis.
- The type of measurements collected (continuous, ordinal data or categorical – see Chapter 3).
- The distribution of the data.
- There should be reasonable variation within the data for each variable.
- Parametric tests can only be applied if the dependent (outcome) variable(s) approximate to the normal distribution.

These criteria form the basis for the set of assumptions that underpins each test. As a reviewer, your main task is to check that the researcher has adhered to the assumptions for each statistical test used.

What determines the 'significance' of a statistical test?

Each statistical test is based on a unique algorithm (mathematical formula or set of computational rules). When this algorithm is applied to the data set, the result is a numerical value called the value of the test statistic. The statistical significance of this value depends on the sample size or 'degrees of freedom'. Statistical significance is indicated by the value of p, as in the following example:

Group A scored higher than group B ($t = 1.8$, df $= 60$, $p \leq 0.05$).

- $t = 1.8$ gives the value of the test statistic, in this case for the independent t test.
- df = degrees of freedom. In the case of the t test, df $= n - 2$, where n is the number of subjects included in the analysis. So df $= 60$ indicates that the total number of subjects is 62 (note that this may be less than the original sample if there are missing data).
- p = the probability that there is *no* difference between groups A and B (the null hypothesis).

We explain each of these aspects in more detail below.

The test statistic

Each statistical test is allocated a unique letter (t, r, F or whatever), followed by a number or value. This letter signifies to the reviewer which test that has been used (though we refer in subsequent chapters to some exceptions where the results have been transformed into a different format for ease of interpretation).

Prior to the advent of computerised data analysis, statistical test results were calculated by hand and the statistical significance of the test statistic was determined using statistical tables. Nowadays, the whole calculation is done on computer using a statistical package such as SPSS (Statistical Package for the Social Sciences).

The researcher enters the data into the computer and selects which statistical test to use. The test algorithm is applied to the data and the result given as the value of the test statistic (e.g. $t = 1.8$).

Statistical packages ensure that the calculation is totally reliable. But they rely on the researcher to input the data correctly and select the correct test. The computer cannot compensate for mistakes in data entry or instruction, hence the term 'garbage in, garbage out'. The reviewer should be able to spot potential errors and statistical tables, as we will show, remain a valuable tool in this process.

Degrees of freedom (df)

This term can seem intimidating, but it reflects an important concept in statistics. Statisticians are keen to avoid Type I error (incorrectly classifying a result as statistically significant). Therefore for each analysis, they reduce the number of observations or categories to those that are free to vary once the totals are known. The number of observations or categories left following this adjustment is referred to as the 'degrees of freedom (df)'.

Explaining degrees of freedom

Suppose that 5 people each answer a satisfaction question using a four-point scale, and suppose their total score is 14 (see Table 10.1).

Since the final running total must equal the grand total, it is clear that the score for participant no. 5 can only be 4. Thus the value of the last entry is not free to vary if the grand total is known. Therefore the degrees of freedom (df) $= n - 1 = 4$, where $n = 5$ is the total number of observations included in the analysis.

Table 10.1 Explaining degrees of freedom ($n = 5$)

Participant number	Score	Running total
1	2	2
2	3	5
3	1	6
4	4	10
5	?	?
Grand total	14	

This statistical correction has most impact where the sample size is small.

A similar rationale is applied to degrees of freedom for categorical data. In the example of a contingency table given in Table 10.2, values for Group B are not free to vary once the number of 'yes' responses for Group A and the totals for groups and responses are known. Generally for contingency tables df = (number of rows − 1) × (number of columns − 1). Table 10.2 illustrates that the degrees of freedom for a 2 (categories) × 2 (responses) table are (2 − 1) × (2 − 1) = 1.

Table 10.2 Degrees of freedom in a contingency table

	Group A	Group B	Total
Yes	30	?	50
No	?	?	50
Total	50	50	100

Values for each cell marked ? can be calculated once the totals are known and are therefore 'not free to vary'. Of the four shaded cells that contain the results, only one result is free to vary, hence df = 1.

Value of *p* and statistical significance

The value of *p* gives the probability that there is *no* difference or *no* association. The default value of *p* considered to be statistically significant is $p \leq 0.05$. It indicates a 95% likelihood that there really is a difference or association. A comprehensive explanation of probability is given in Chapter 9.

One tail or two?

It is essential that each test of probability matches the hypothesis: a directional hypothesis is tested using a one-tailed test of probability, while a non-directional hypothesis is tested using a two-tailed test of probability. You will find a detailed explanation in Chapter 9. It will affect the statistical significance of the research results.

Using statistical tables

Where inadequate statistical information is given by the researcher or the reviewer suspects an error, it is useful to check the results using a set of standard statistical tables, available in any basic textbook on statistics or the internet.

A statistical table gives a series of 'critical values' for a particular test statistic. There are cut-off points that determine the thresholds for different levels of statistical significance, depending on the sample size (*n*) or degrees of freedom (df), and the nature of the hypothesis (one- or two-tailed). Table 10.3 illustrates how this can be applied.

Table 10.3 Extract of statistical table for the t test, with interpretation

Column of values of t if $p = 0.05$, one-tailed

Column of values of t if $p = 0.05$, two-tailed

df	Level of significance for a one-tailed test					
	.10 (ns)	.05	.025	.01	.005	.0005
	Level of significance for a two-tailed test					
	.20 (ns)	.10 (ns)	.05	.02	.01	.001
20	1.325	1.725	2.086	2.528	2.845	3.850
25	1.316	1.708	2.060	2.485	2.787	3.725
30	1.310	1.697	2.042	2.457	2.750	3.646
40	1.303	1.684	2.021	2.423	2.704	3.551
60	1.296	1.671	2.000	2.390	2.660	3.460
120	1.289	1.658	1.980	2.358	2.617	3.373
Infinity	1.282	1.645	1.960	2.326	2.576	3.291

Row containing critical values of t if df = 60 (n = 62)

t = 1.8 achieves statistical significance using a one-tailed test of probability

A minimum value of t = 2 is required to achieve statistical significance using a two-tailed test of probability

The test result is given as (t = 1.8, df 60, $p < 0.05$), but it is not clear if a one-tailed or two-tailed test of probability was applied.

Using the statistical table for critical values of t, it is possible to verify that a one-tailed test of probability must have been used. The result would not have been statistically significant had a two-tailed test of probability been applied.

How are research results presented?

Statistical results may be presented in the form of text, or are contained within a table, graph or forest plot. Unfortunately, there is no generally accepted or standard approach.

Text presentation

The following are alternative examples of presentation:

1 As predicted, group A scored higher than group B (t = 2.1, df 36, one-tailed $p \leq 0.05$).
2 As predicted, group A scored higher than group B ($t(36) = 2.1$, $p \leq 0.05$).
3 Contentment increased with income ($r = 0.5$, $n = 136$, $p < 0.001$).

Example 1 gives statistical information in full.

Example 2 gives the degrees of freedom in brackets. A one-tailed test is implied by the term 'as predicted'.

In Example 3, correlation results are given using n, rather than df. In this example, it is not clear if the value of p is one-tailed or two-tailed. It is necessary to check in the Method section to see which test of probability was applied. If not stated, it is necessary to check the result against the statistical tables for r.

Tables of results

These are usually used where a series of comparisons are made, as in Table 10.4.

Table 10.4 Example of table of full results

Dependent variable	Mean (sd) group 1 $n = 30$	Mean (sd) group 2 $n = 30$	t	one-tailed p
Well-being	26.5 (1.2)	23.5 (0.8)	2	0.05

Values of t can easily be calculated provided the means, standard deviations and values of n are given (see Chapter 11), so it is permissible to omit the value of t and abbreviate the results, as in Table 10.5.

Table 10.5 Abbreviated table of group means

Dependent variable	Mean (sd) group 1 $n = 30$	Mean (sd) group 2 $n = 30$
Variable 1	26.5 (1.2)	23.5 (0.8)*[†]
Variable 2	30.1 (2.1)	31.5 (2.3)
Variable 3	34.2 (2.3)	33.5 (2.2)

*$p \leq 0.05$
[†] Independent t test

In Table 10.5, standard deviations are given in brackets, the statistical test used and different levels of statistical significance identified using a reference system explained underneath the table.

Graphs and matrices

Results that include both within-group and between-group comparisons (see Chapter 14 on ANOVA), are sometimes illustrated using a graph, as in Figure 1.5 in Chapter 1.

Correlations are often presented in the form of a matrix – see Table 15.2 (Chapter 15).

Forest plots

Results of clinical trials usually include confidence intervals giving the range of values within which the true value is likely to be found in 95% or 99% of the target population. Confidence intervals are increasingly presented in the form of a forest plot. Figure 10.1 illustrates two alternative forms.

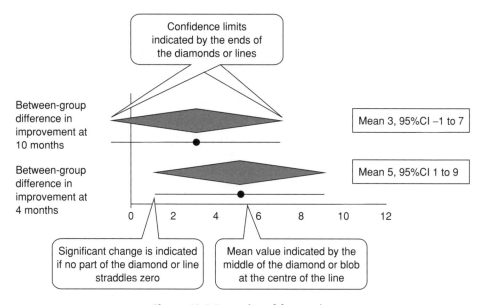

Figure 10.1 Examples of forest plot

Other forms of presentation

Other forms of presentation include the correlation matrix (see Chapter 15), bar charts and pie charts (Chapter 5).

Checklist for review

Figure 10.2 summarises a systematic approach that is helpful when reviewing statistical results.

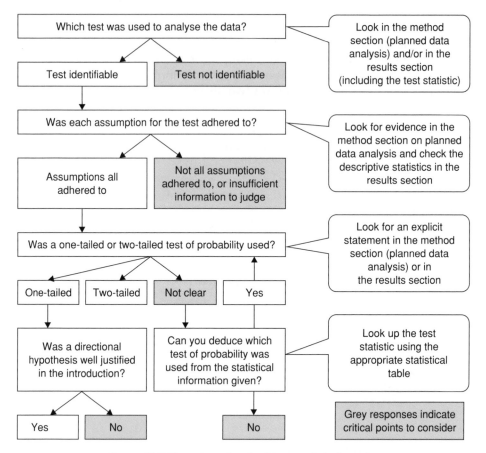

Figure 10.2 Flow chart for checking statistical results

Further reading

A free source of information about various statistical tests (available at the time of writing) can be found at http://www.stat-help.com/notes.html.

The following books are aimed at those wanting to analyse data, and are accessible and informative:

Dancey, C.P. and Reidy, J. (2007) *Statistics without Maths for Psychology: Using SPSS for Windows,* 4th edition. London: Pearson Prentice Hall.

Field, A. (2009) *Discovering Statistics Using SPSS,* 3rd edition. London: Sage.

Jaeger, R.M. (1983) *Statistics: Spectator Sport,* 2nd edition. Newbury Park, CA: Sage.

11 Comparing Two Independent (Unrelated) Groups:
Independent (unrelated) *t* test, Mann–Whitney *U* test and Contingency analysis – Fisher's exact test and chi-square test

---

KEY QUESTIONS

- What sorts of research questions or hypotheses are answered using these tests?
- What assumptions need to be met for the results of these tests to be valid?
- How should I interpret the results of these tests?

Purpose

The tests of group difference (group comparison) in this chapter are designed to test for statistical differences between a single set of measurements taken from two independent or unrelated groups. In health care research, their main uses are:

- in a clinical trial, to compare baseline measurements between one experimental and one control group (see the example in Chapter 1);
- in surveys, to compare measurements taken from two separate groups sampled from the same population (see the example in Chapter 2).

Type of hypothesis tested

The hypothesis predicts a difference between two groups. We illustrate this using an imaginary study to explore differences in fidgeting between boys and girls. Note that all statistical tests test the null hypothesis that there is *no* difference, in this case between boys and girls. The smaller the probability that there is no difference (the smaller the value of *p*), the greater the probability that there really *is* a difference (between boys and girls).

Example

Hypothesis: boys fidget more than girls
This hypothesis provides the following information:
1. The groups to be compared are boys and girls.
2. The dependent variable is fidgeting. We have selected two measures:
   • Parental Report Scale of Fidgeting;
   • direct observation score of attention span.
3. The hypothesis is directional:
   • boys will score higher on the fidget scale than girls;
   • boys will return a lower attention score than girls.

You may find if helpful to draw up a chart, similar to the one in Table 11.1, to help you to organise your critique:

Table 11.1 Guide to critique for tests of group difference (two groups)

Dependent variable	Groups			
Fidgeting	Boys vs girls (B vs G)			
Dependent measures	H_0	Test used	Assumptions checked?	Test result
Fidget scale	$B > G$			
Attention score	$B < G$			

H_0 is the null hypothesis.

How do I check that the appropriate test was used?

In the final 'Analysis' part of their Method section, the researchers should state either the exact names of the test(s), or if a parametric or nonparametric test was used. The key task for the reviewer is to check that the set of assumptions for each test has been adhered to (see Table 11.2).

Table 11.2 Assumptions that determine which test should be used to compare two groups

ASSUMPTIONS	t test	Mann–Whitney U test	Fisher exact test Chi-square test
Sampling	The two groups must be sampled from the same population. The data must be obtained from two separate (unrelated) groups of participants.		
Measurement of the dependent variable	Continuous, interval scale	Interval or ordinal scale	Number counts in discrete categories
Distribution of the dependent variable	Normal distribution only	Any distribution, provided there is reasonable spread of data across the range	Fisher exact test if the measure has two categories Chi-square if minimum cell size requirement is achieved[a]

[a] For 2 (groups) × 2 (response categories) 10 expected observations are required in each cell. For more response categories, there must be at least 5 expected observations in each cell (as explained later in this chapter).

The fidget study 1: testing for demographic differences
Before comparing boys and girls, it is important to check that the groups are demographically similar. Younger children tend to fidget more than older children, so age difference may confound difference in fidgeting.

> **Hypothesis:** There is an age difference between boys and girls in the study.
> **Sampling criteria:** The children were sampled from the same nurseries and schools.
> **Dependent measure:** Age.

The test of group difference used depends on the measure of age:

- If age is measured in years, a *t* test would be used, provided the data for both groups approximate to the normal distribution.
- If age is measured using four or more sequential age bands (e.g. 3–4, 5–6, 7–10, 12–15), the data are ordinal and the **Mann–Whitney *U* test** would be used.
- If age is recorded using three discrete age groups (e.g. 3–5, 6–9, 10–16), the **chi-square test** would be used, provided the sample size was large enough.
- If age is recorded as two (dichotomous) age groups (e.g. 3–8, 9–16), the **Fisher exact test** or chi-square test would be used.

The fidget study 2: testing the hypothesis that boys fidget more than girls
Fidgeting was measured using a six-point 'fidget scale' from 1 'never' to 6 'all the time'. This is an ordinal scale, so the appropriate test of comparison is the **Mann–Whitney *U* test**.

Attention was measured by the length of time the child maintained focused attention on a task during a 10-minute period of direct observation. This is a continuous, interval scale so the appropriate test of comparison is the *t* test, provided the data set for each group conforms to the normal distribution. It is important to check that the data for attention was not skewed (see Chapter 4).

The independent or unrelated *t* test (also referred to as Student's *t* test)

The independent *t* test is used to compare mean values taken from two independent groups, provided the distributions are 'normal'. This is illustrated in Figure 11.1, where irregularities in the distribution have been smoothed out to give two similar normal distribution curves.

Conceptually, the result of the *t* test depends on the extent of separation between the means, taking account of the proportion of overlap (similarity) in the distributions (the grey area).

Assumptions of the independent or unrelated *t* test

The independent *t* test relies on the following assumptions, and the reviewer must check that they have been adhered to:

1. Data from individuals in one group are not paired with, or related to, data from the other group.

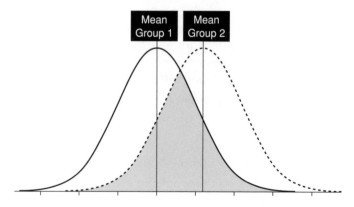

Figure 11.1 Comparison of two means in normally distributed data

2. The dependent variable is measured using a continuous scale that has 11 or more equidistant intervals (e.g. points on the scale 0, 1, 2, ..., 10). If not, the Mann–Whitney U test should be used.

3. Look at the descriptive statistics at the beginning of the results section. Does the distribution approximate to the normal distribution? (See Chapter 4 for indicators.) If not, the Mann–Whitney U test should be used.

4. Are the standard deviations for each group similar? (This is termed 'homogeneity of variance'.) If the standard deviations appear different, look to see if the researchers have tested for a significant difference between the standard deviations using Levene's test for equality of error variance. If the result of this test is given as $p \leq 0.05$ it means the standard deviations are statistically different and a 'separate variance' version of the t test must be reported.

The calculation of *t*

Provided the size of, and standard deviations for, each group are similar, the reviewer can easily check the result of a t test using the following formula:

$$t = \frac{\text{mean (group 1)} - \text{mean (group 2)}}{\text{pooled standard deviation (sd)}}$$

Example

In the fidget study:

- Total sample size (boys + girls) = 62.
- Degrees of freedom (df) for the t test = $n - 2 = 60$.
- Hypothesis is directional (boys will show lower attention time than girls).
- Mean (girls) – mean (boys) = 5.1.
- sd (boys) = 1.9; sd (girls) = 1.7, therefore mean sd = 1.8 (approx).

Therefore

$$t = \frac{5.1}{1.8} = 2.8.$$

Presentation of results

The results can be presented in the form of table or text, for example:

The results for attention span support the hypothesis that boys fidget more than girls ($t = 2.8$, df 60, one-tailed $p < 0.005$).

Table 11.3 contrasts two ways of presenting this statistical information in tabular form. The inclusion of the t statistic is desirable, but not essential if group means and standard deviations are provided.

Table 11.3 Group comparisons in tables

Dependent variable	Mean (sd) boys ($n = 31$)	Mean (sd) girls ($n = 31$)	t	p
Fidget score	7.0 (1.7)	12.1 (1.9)	2.8	<0.005

Dependent variable	Mean (sd) group A ($n = 31$)	Mean (sd) group B ($n = 31$)
Fidget scale	7.0 (1.7)	12.1 (1.9)***

*** $p < 0.005$

Mean
Standard deviation
Level of probability interpreted below

Checking the value of p

Provided the value of t is known, it is possible to use a set of statistical tables to check the value of p (see Chapter 10).

In Table 11.4, each shaded cell contains a 'critical value' of t. This is the minimum value of t to achieve significance for a minimum value of df (which is $n - 2$). For example, if $t = 2.8$ and df $= 62$ (i.e. $n = 60$), it is possible to confirm that for a one-tailed test, $p < 0.005$ (the likelihood that there is no difference between the group means is less than 5:1000).

Jellesma et al. (2008) compared reactions to peer relationships between boys and girls. Non-directional research questions included: 'Are girls better at emotional communication skills than boys?' The findings (page 2200) are stated as follows:

Although there also seemed to be a trend for girls scoring higher on emotion communication skill, boys and girls did not significantly differ on this variable, t (568) = 1.7, $p = 0.07$.

Example

In the above example, it is not clear if a one-tailed or a two-tailed test of significance was used. The extract from the statistical table in Table 11.5 shows that a value of $t \geq 1.6$ would achieve significance had a directional test of probability been applied (one-tailed $p = 0.05$), but not using a non-directional test, in line with the research question (two-tailed $p = 0.1$, not significant).

Table 11.4 Extract from statistical table for *t*, highlighting one-tailed probability associated with a *t* value of at least 2.7 and *n* = 62

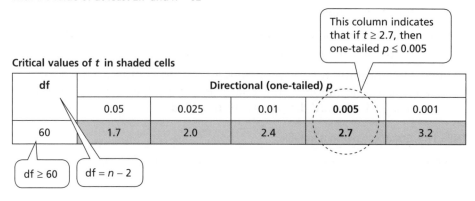

This column indicates that if $t \geq 2.7$, then one-tailed $p \leq 0.005$

Critical values of *t* in shaded cells

df	Directional (one-tailed) *p*				
	0.05	0.025	0.01	**0.005**	0.001
60	1.7	2.0	2.4	**2.7**	3.2

df ≥ 60   df = *n* − 2

Table 11.5 Extract from statistical table for the *t* test for large sample size

Each column gives the level of probability associated with nearest 'Critical' value of *t*

df	Directional (one-tailed) *p*				
	0.05	0.025	0.01	0.005	0.0005
	Non-directional (two-tailed) *p*				
	0.1 (ns)	0.05	0.02	0.01	0.001
120+	**1.6**	2.0	2.3	2.6	3.3

ns = not significant.

The Mann–Whitney *U* test

Rather confusingly, this is now often referred to as the **Wilcoxon–Mann–Whitney *U* test** in recognition of the role played by Wilcoxon in its development (not to be confused with the Wilcoxon signed rank test for repeated measures (see Chapter 13).

The Mann–Whitney test is the nonparametric equivalent of the independent *t* test. Instead of comparing group means, it compares the ranked scores for each group (see Chapter 5 for details of ranking).

Assumptions of the Mann–Whitney *U* test

There are few assumptions for this nonparametric test. It is safe to use if the dependent variable is ordinal (see Chapter 3) or interval, regardless of distribution and is appropriate where the sample sizes are small or unequal.

Interpreting the Mann–Whitney U test

Unlike the t test, the Mann–Whitney test compares the raw data, not the group means, so it is not possible to check the calculation. However, researchers often give the mean rank score for each group to give some idea of group difference.

Comparing fidgeting using the Parental Report scale

The data in Table 11.6 are based on comparisons between 8 boys and 7 girls, based on the ordinal fidget scale. Because there is a total of 15 children, ranked scores will range from 1 to 15.

Table 11.6 Actual and ranked fidget scores with girls' scores in bold

15 fidget scores are placed in ascending order

Fidget scale score	1	1	2	2	3	3	3	3	3	4	4	4	5	5
Rank score	1.5	1.5	3.5	3.5	6	6	6	8.5	8.5	11	11	11	13.5	13.5

Note how children scoring 2 lie 3rd and 4th in the hierarchy, so share the rank score of 3.5

- Total rank score (girls) = 1.5 + 1.5 + 3.5 + 6 + 6 + 6 + 11 = 35.5
- Mean rank (girls) = 35.5 ÷ 7 = 5.07
- Total rank score (boys) = 3.5 + 8.5 + 8.5 + 11 + 11 + 13.5 + 13.5 + 15 = 84.5
- Mean rank (boys) = 84.5 ÷ 8 = 10.6

This result suggests a difference between boys and girls, but is it statistically significant?

Example

Interpreting the results

Statistical tables for U (see Table 11.7) confirm that the value of U (48.5) lies within the range of numbers (6 to 50) that *fail* to achieve significance with sample sizes of 7 and 8.

If either sample size exceeds 20, the results are transformed into a **z score** for ease of interpretation. The z score is a standardised score that represents the number of standard deviations the value of U lies away from the point of no difference.

If the hypothesis is non-directional (two-tailed), a critical z score of at least ±1.96 indicates a statistically significant difference between the two groups (two-tailed $p \leq 0.05$).

Table 11.7 Extract from critical values of *U* for group sizes 7 and 8

N boys/N girls	6	7	8
7	3–39	4–45	6–50
8	4–44	6–50	7–57
9	5–49	7–56	9–63

Values of *U* for 8 boys and 7 girls. Values within this range of numbers **fail** to achieve significance

If the hypothesis is directional, a critical *z* score of at least ±1.64 indicates a statistically significant difference between the two groups (one-tailed $p \leq 0.05$).

Contingency tables and contingency analysis

Contingency analysis is based on a 'contingency table' that contains a series of observations in mutually exclusive cells or categories (see the example in Table 11.8).

The dependent measure must be based on frequency counts (the number of people or observations in each category) and not on measurement scores or values.

Fallis and Fricke (2002) sought to examine the accuracy of health information contained on authorised versus unauthorised web pages. Authorisation was indicated by the logo of the Health On the Net Foundation's Code of Conduct (HON code). The hypothesis was that there would be more errors in unauthorised web pages (i.e. those where the HON code logo was not displayed).

The results are given in the form of a 2 (rows) × 2 (columns) contingency table in which there are four possible response categories or 'cells' (Table 11.8).

Table 11.8 Contingency table showing accuracy of web pages according to display of HON code (from Fallis and Fricke 2002: 76)

	Web page is more accurate	Web page is less accurate
HON code logo is displayed	11	3
HON code logo is not displayed	39	47

Each cell contains a count of the number of observations (web pages) recorded in that category

There are two tests that can be used to analyse group differences using frequency measurements:

- Fisher's exact test is used only for a 2 (groups) × 2 (categories) contingency table, particularly if the sample size is small.
- The chi-square (χ^2) test may be used where there are two or more groups and the dependent variable consists of two or more categories.

Fisher's exact test

This test is widely used to compare two groups where the dependent variable consists of a mutually exclusive frequency count such as 'present/absent', 'improved/not improved', 'cured/not cured'. It may be used in RCTs to compare one intervention with one control group where the outcome can be classified as either successful or unsuccessful.

Assumption of Fisher's exact test

There are two separate, randomly selected groups and the dependent variable consists only of two mutually exclusive categories.

Presentation of results

There is no test statistic associated with Fisher's exact test. Instead the result is given as an exact probability (value of p). The value of p refers to the probability that there is *no* discrepancy between the recorded (observed) values and the values expected if the observations are proportionate to the numbers in each group (see example in the next section).

Chi-square test

Chi-square (χ^2) is used to determine if there is a discrepancy between the distribution of the actual observations (the observed values) for each group and the values that would be expected if the data were distributed proportionately (the expected values).

Assumptions of chi-square

1. The dependent variable is categorical.
2. Each participant or observation can be recorded in only one category or cell in the contingency table.
3. There is a minimum response size requirement:
   - For a 2 × 2 table, it is generally recommended that there should be a minimum 'expected' frequency of 10 in each cell. If not, Fisher's exact test should be used.
   - If the dependent variable consists of more than two categories, at least 80% of cells must contain a minimum 'expected' frequency of 5. No cell should contain zero observations. (See below for an explanation of expected frequency.)

Understanding chi-square

Chi-square is easy to calculate from a table of data.

1. The expected values for each cell are calculated, based on the ratio of the totals for each row and column.
2. The ratio of discrepancy between each actual (observed) and the expected value is calculated (see the example in Table 11.9).
3. These discrepancy values are summed to give the value for chi-square.

Table 11.9 illustrates the differences between observed and expected values in the Fallis and Fricke (2002) study, together with an example of how to calculate an expected value.

Table 11.9 Contingency table showing observed and expected values, with example of expected value calculation (from Fallis and Fricke 2002)

	Web page accurate	Web page not accurate	Total
HON code displayed	observed 11 / 7 expected	observed 3 / 7 expected	14
No HON code displayed	observed 39 / 43 expected	observed 47 / 43 expected	86
Total	50	50	100

Expected number of inaccurate pages if code not displayed = 50 (inaccurate) × 86 (no code displayed) ÷ 100 (total sample) = 43

For those who are interested, the formula for chi-square is:

$$\chi^2 = \sum \frac{(\text{observed value} - \text{expected value})^2}{\text{expected value}}$$

where $\sum$ means 'sum of'. In the example from Table 11.9:

$$\chi^2 = \frac{(11-7)^2}{7} + \frac{(3-7)^2}{7} + \frac{(39-43)^2}{43} + \frac{(47-43)^2}{43} = 5.3.$$

The results would be stated in the following type of format:

Accurate websites were more likely than inaccurate websites to display the HON code ($\chi^2 = 5.3$, df 1, $p \leq 0.05$).

Degrees of freedom in chi-square

The degrees of freedom (df) for chi-square are calculated by:

df = (number of rows − 1) × (number of columns − 1).

This information enables the reviewer to check the number of categories that comprise the dependent variable. For example, if df = 2 and the number of groups to be compared is two, the dependent variable must consist of three categories:

(2 groups − 1) × (3 categories − 1) = 2.

The most common problem associated with the use of chi-square is the failure to achieve an adequate sample size. As the number of categories increase, the sample size must increase to ensure that the 'rule of 5' expected observations per cell can be met.

Summary

The following tests are used to compare two unrelated groups:

- the independent *t* test, a parametric test, if the dependent measure is continuous and approximates to the normal distribution;
- the Mann–Whitney *U* test, a nonparametric test, if the dependent measure is ordinal or continuous – appropriate for small samples and odd distibutions;
- Fisher's exact test, if the dependent measure is dichotomous;
- chi-square, if the dependent measure consists of frequency counts in mutually exclusive, unrelated categories and the minimum sample size requirement is met.

Further reading

Pett, M.A. (1977) *Nonparametric Statistics for Health Care Research: Statistics for Small Samples and Unusual Distributions*. Thousand Oaks, CA: Sage.

12 Comparing Three or More Independent (Unrelated) Groups:
One-way ANOVA, Kruskal–Wallis test and Chi-square test

KEY QUESTIONS

- What sorts of research questions or hypotheses are answered using these tests?
- What assumptions need to be met for the results of these tests to be valid?
- How should I interpret the results of these tests?

Introduction

The principles for these tests are similar to those described in Chapter 11, except that they are designed to test for differences between three or more independent or unrelated groups. For example:

- in an RCT, a comparison of baseline measurements from one experimental group compared to two or more control groups;
- in a survey, a comparison of well-being between those from three different types of locality (e.g. urban, suburban, rural) or those described according to five different social class backgrounds.

You will find it easier to understand this chapter if you have familiarised yourself with the simpler tests explained in Chapter 11.

Comparing three or more groups

Table 12.1 gives an overview of the assumptions that underpin the tests outlined in this chapter. The main task of the reviewer is to ensure that the researchers have adhered to these.

One-way analysis of variance (ANOVA or *F* test)

One-way analysis of variance (ANOVA) is an extension of the *t* test to compare more than two groups (see Figure 12.1). It is sometimes referred to as the *F* test because the test statistic is labelled *F*.

Table 12.1 Checklist of assumptions for tests of comparison for three or more groups

ASSUMPTIONS	One-way analysis of variance (ANOVA)	Kruskal–Wallis one-way ANOVA by ranks	Chi-square test
Sampling	Groups must be sampled from the same population		
Number of dependent variables	One		
Measurement of the dependent variable	Continuous, interval scale	Interval or ordinal scale	Discrete categories
Distribution of the dependent variable	Normal. Standard deviations must be similar for each group	Any distribution with reasonable variation across the range	At least 5 expected observations[a] in at least 80% of cells range

[a] See Table 11.9 for an explanation of the difference between observed and expected observations.

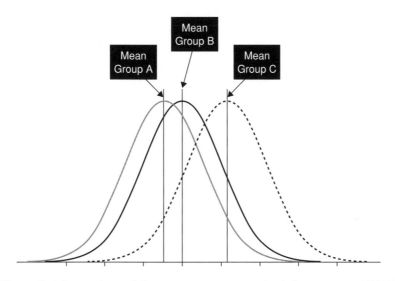

Figure 12.1 Comparison of three group means as a basis for one-way ANOVA

In Figure 12.1, it appears that the means for groups A and B are similar, while the mean for group C is different. ANOVA tests whether or not any of the mean differences (AB, AC, BC) is statistically significant, taking into account the amount of overlap in the distribution of the data.

Assumptions of one-way ANOVA

- There are three or more groups to be compared.
- The dependent measure is continuous and the data for each group approximate to the normal distribution.

- The standard deviations for each group are similar. This assumption is referred to as 'homogeneity of variance'.

Interpreting the results of ANOVA

The results of ANOVA contain important items of information, given in one of the following equivalent ways:

- $F(2,117) = 4.0, p \leq 0.05$
- $F_{2,117} = 4.0, p \leq 0.05$
- $F = 4.0$, df = 2, 117, $p \leq 0.05$.

We interpret these as follows:

- F indicates that ANOVA was the statistical test used.
- The numbers 2 and 117 represent two sets of degrees of freedom: between groups and within groups. The first, 2, which is the number of groups minus 1, indicates that three groups were compared. The second, 117, which is the total number of observations minus the number of groups, indicates that a total of 120 complete sets of data were included in the analysis.
- 4.0 is the value of the F statistic.
- $p \leq 0.05$ indicates that the result is statistically significant, assuming a significance level of $\alpha = 0.05$.

Example

Jellesma et al. (2008) wanted to compare the effects of different types of friendship on somatic complaints. They divided the children into three separate groups:

- children with a mutual best friend (group A);
- children who failed to nominate a best friend (group B);
- children with an unreciprocated best friend (group C).

Analysis of variance was used to compare the number of somatic complaints recorded for each of these three groups. The results reported (page 2200) as follows:

The groups did not differ on somatic complaints, F(2,605) = 0.86, ns.

$F = 0.86$ gives the value of the F statistic;

(2,605) = degrees of freedom (between groups, within groups), which tells the reviewer that three groups were compared and data from a total of 608 children were included in the analysis (out of the original sample size of 688). The result was not statistically significant (ns).

Using statistical tables for F (see Table 12.2), it is possible to confirm that the value of F (0.86) was well short of the critical value (3.1) required to achieve statistical significance for the specified sample size.

Table 12.2 Extract from table of critical values for F

df (between groups) groups – 1	df (within groups) n-groups					
	20	30	40	50	100	1000
2	3.5	3.3	3.2	3.1	3.1	3.0

Critical values of F associated with $p = 0.05$ are given in the shaded cells

Analysis of covariance (ANCOVA)

ANCOVA is identical to ANOVA in terms of its assumptions and presentation of results. The key difference is that it is used to control for baseline or demographic differences between groups that might confound the result.

For example, if differences between a demographic variable such as age is thought likely to confound a study of group differences in well-being, ANCOVA would be used to hold the covariate, age, constant during the analysis. Thus, statistical control is used to eliminate any biasing effect of age.

Post hoc planned tests of comparison (pairwise multiple comparisons)

ANOVA and ANCOVA identify that there is a statistical difference between the group means, but it does not identify the source of difference (in Figure 12.1, A versus B; A versus C; B versus C). Post hoc pairwise tests of comparison are used to ascertain the precise location of group differences.

Post hoc comparisons are similar to conducting a series of t tests between each group, but are more cautious. They are termed 'post hoc' (literally 'after the event') because they are only used after a significant value of F has been obtained. There is a choice of tests which include:

- Tukey's HSD (honestly significant difference);
- Scheffé's test;
- Least significant difference test – this is equivalent to doing a series of pairwise t tests.

There are others – every statistician appears to have a favourite!

In the study by Jellesma et al. (2008), ANCOVA showed a significant effect of classroom status on social anxiety, after controlling for the effect of gender (the covariate). Classroom status (the independent variable) consisted of five groups to be compared: popular, rejected, neglected, controversial and average. The dependent measure was social anxiety.

A Tukey–Kramer post hoc procedure was used to compare social anxiety between the five groups. This showed that, when compared to the neglected and rejected children, those classified as 'controversial' reported less social anxiety.

Example

Why bother with ANOVA? Why not just compare each pair of means in turn? Some researchers do this by using a series of *t* tests, but it is actually a form of cheating. This is because multiple tests of comparison inflate the significance of any differences and are more susceptible to Type I error (false positive findings).

Kruskal–Wallis one-way analysis of variance by ranks

This is the nonparametric equivalent of one-way ANOVA. Like one-way ANOVA, it is used to compare three or more independent groups or samples. It is used in preference to ANOVA when the dependent variable is ordinal or fails to approximate to the normal distribution.

The Kruskal–Wallis test is used to detect a statistically different difference between the rank scores of any of the groups. The formula is of little use to the reviewer who has no access to the raw data. Similar to the Mann–Whitney *U* test (Chapter 11), it is based on group differences in the mean rank values for the dependent variable, rather than the actual mean values (see Chapter 5 for an explanation of rank values). Conceptually, when the difference between the average rank scores for any of the groups is too large to be attributable to sampling error, a significant difference between the groups suspected.

The Kruskal–Wallis test statistic, denoted by *H*, is calculated when each group is no more than 20 strong. When larger groups are compared, the χ^2 (chi-square) statistic is calculated instead (see Chapter 11; we refer to it again in the next section of this chapter).

As with ANOVA, the Kruskal–Wallis test does not identify the precise sources of group differences, so once a significant result is obtained, a series of Mann–Whitney *U* tests is used to locate these.

Assumptions of the Kruskal–Wallis test

The only assumptions are the following:

1. There are three or more independent groups to be compared.
2. The dependent measurements may be either interval or ordinal, but must have data distributed across at least four scale points.

Contingency analysis: the chi-square test

The principles of the chi-square test were described in Chapter 11 and are exactly the same whether the comparison is between two, three or more independent groups, using a dependent variable that has two, three or more independent categories.

Assumptions of the chi-square test

1. The data must be based on frequency counts (number of participants or observations in each separate category).
2. An observation or individual can be counted in only one category or cell.

3. There must be at least five expected observations in at least 80% of cells and no cell should have zero observations. (See Chapter 11 for explanation).

Problems associated with chi-square

The main problem is the need for a large sample size to ensure at least 5 expected observations in at least 80% of cells. Unless the distribution has been reasonably accurately predicted in advance, a very large sample size may be required to ensure that this requirement is achieved (see Chapter 8).

If a researcher finds that their data fail to meet the requirement for at least 5 expected observations in 80% of cells, or if there is a cell with no observations, they have the option to collapse two or more categories together so that the assumption is met. The reviewer must judge if this is acceptable from a theoretical perspective and does not merely represent an attempt to find a significant result at all costs.

Summary

The following tests are used to compare three or more unrelated groups:

- One-way ANOVA, a parametric test, if the dependent measure is continuous and approximates to the normal distribution, and the group distributions are statistically comparable (homogeneity of variance)

- Kruskal–Wallis, a nonparametric test, if the dependent measure is ordinal or the assumptions for ANOVA cannot be met.

- Chi-square, if the dependent measure consists of frequency counts in mutually exclusive, unrelated categories and the minimum sample size requirement is met.

13 Comparing Two Sets of Related Data: Matched Pairs or Single-Sample Repeated Measures — Related (paired) *t* test, Wilcoxon signed rank test, Sign test and McNemar's test

KEY QUESTIONS

- What sorts of research questions or hypotheses are answered using these tests?
- What assumptions need to be met for the results of these tests to be valid?
- How should I interpret the results of these tests?

Introduction

These tests are all designed to test for differences between the means of repeated measurements taken at two points in time from a single group, or for a paired set of measurements taken from two groups. For example:

- to test for improvement in well-being in the same group of people before and after a change in lifestyle has taken place;
- to compare quality of life from a set of data collected from pairs of individuals with and without a specific medical condition, matched on demographic variables.

Test assumptions

The test assumptions relate primarily to the type of data collected, as shown in Table 13.1.

Example

In Chapter 11 we discussed an imaginary study to compare fidgeting in boys and girls. Our hypothesis was that boys fidget more than girls.

In this study, an identical set of measurements was taken from 20 pairs of boy/girl siblings, to control for the effects of social background. The dependent variables were:

1. Attention-span score, based on the number of seconds the child is recorded as fidgeting during a 10-minute period of observation.

2. A fidget scale consisting of a six-point ordinal scale of frequency (from never to all the time).

An additional categorical measure was recorded: whether or not the child was labelled by the parent as a fidget (yes/no).

   In the following sections, we use these three types of data to illustrate the statistical tests available.

Table 13.1 Assumptions that determine which test should be used to compare matched or related data

ASSUMPTIONS	Related *t* test	Wilcoxon signed rank test	McNemar's test
Sampling	An identical set of measurements is taken either from related or matched pairs of individuals, or from the same individual at different points in time		
Measurement of the dependent variable	Continuous, interval scale	Interval or ordinal scale	Discrete categories
Distribution of the dependent variable	Normal distribution only	Any distribution, provided there is reasonable spread of data across the range	Reasonable spread of data across the categories

Related (paired or correlated) *t* test

The related *t* test is based on paired difference scores, in this case 'boy minus girl' attention-span scores. The value of *t* is interpreted the same as for the independent *t* test (see Chapter 11) and the results are presented in the same way:

   Boys fidget more than girls ($t = 2.6$, df $= 19$, one-tailed $p \leq 0.01$)

Note that the degrees of freedom for the related *t* test are $n - 1$, where n is the total sample size (boys plus girls).

Assumptions of the related (paired) *t* test:

1. The data must consist of pairs of scores.

2. The data are continuous and approximate to the normal distribution.

Wilcoxon signed rank test

This test is the nonparametric equivalent of the related *t* test, used to compare data taken from the same group on two separate occasions, or data from matched samples. The calculation is based on differences between the rank positions (see Chapters 5 and 10) of the measurements for each pair, rather than changes in the actual values.

- The test statistic is given as W or W_{obs} for a sample size of 20 or less.
- Where the paired sample size is greater than 20, the results are transformed to a z score. The z score represents the number of standard deviations away from zero difference between groups. A score of $z \geq 1.96$ is statistically significant, $p \leq 0.05$, for a two-tailed test, while a score of $z \geq 1.64$ is statistically significant, $p \leq 0.05$, for a one-tailed test.

Assumptions of the Wilcoxon signed rank test:

1. The data must consist of pairs of scores.
2. The data are either continuous or ordinal.

Sign test

The sign test is a very versatile nonparametric test for matched pairs or repeated measures. It simply measures the direction of difference or change for each individual or pair and establishes the probability that the overall direction of change is biased in one direction. It can be used with continuous, ordinal or dichotomous (positive/negative) data. There are no other assumptions attached to it, though it is a somewhat blunt statistical instrument which lacks statistical power.

McNemar's test

McNemar's test is used to compare a single set of matched pairs or repeated measurements where the dependent variable is dichotomous (consists of two categories). It is often used to test for before–after changes where each participant acts as their own control.

The raw results may be presented in the form of a table (see Table 13.2). The McNemar test is concerned with the shift from positive to negative or vice versa. Only cell A (the number which shifted from negative to positive) and cell D (the number shifted from positive to negative) are of interest since these signify change.

The analysis is based on a variation of chi-square based only on cells A and D. The results are given as the χ^2 statistic with df = 1.

Since chi-square is poor at dealing with small numbers, the binomial test is used if the expected frequency $(A + D) \div 2$ is less than 5. The binomial test is the conceptual equivalent to a series of throws of the dice, measuring the number of times a pair of sixes occur. It is given as an exact probability (value of p).

Table 13.2 Before–after changes used as the basis for calculating a shift in position

	Pre-test negative	Pre-test positive
Post-test positive	Number in cell A	Number in cell B
Post-test negative	Number in cell C	Number in cell D

Summary

The following tests are used to compare two matched or paired groups, or the same measurement collected from the same group on two separate occasions:

- Related *t* test, if the dependent measure approximates to the normal distribution.
- Wilcoxon signed rank test or sign test, if the dependent measure is ordinal or continuous. Appropriate for small samples and odd distributions.
- McNemar test if the dependent measure consists of frequency counts in mutually exclusive, unrelated categories.

14 Complex Group Comparisons: ANOVA and ANCOVA, Friedman two-way ANOVA by ranks and Cochrane Q test

KEY QUESTIONS

- What sorts of research questions or hypotheses are answered using these tests?
- What assumptions need to be met for the results of these tests to be valid?
- How should I interpret the results of these tests?

Introduction

These tests are used to answer more complex research questions. For example, a clinical trial is designed to compare measurements or observations collected from multiple groups at multiple points in time.

The choice of test is guided by the research question and the type of data collected, as shown in Table 14.1.

Table 14.1 Tests for repeated measures

	ANOVA/ANCOVA	Friedman two-way ANOVA by ranks	Cochrane Q test
Purpose	Capable of comparing multiple repeated measures taken from multiple groups	Compares a set of multiple matched groups *or* a set of multiple repeated measures taken from a single group	Compares repeated dichotomous measurements taken from a single group
Measurement and distribution of the dependent (outcome) variable	Continuous, interval scale. Conforms to the normal distribution	Interval or ordinal scale	Dichotomous

Analysis of variance

Analysis of variance (ANOVA) is an extremely flexible statistical test commonly used in clinical trials. It is a parametric test, therefore the dependent measurements must approximate to the normal distribution. We discussed one-way ANOVA in Chapter 12.

Two-way ANOVA is used to compare mean differences between two or more groups under two or more different conditions (the independent variables) using a single continuous outcome (dependent) measure.

Repeated measures ANOVA is used to compare mean differences on a single continuous outcome measure taken from a single group at three or more different points in time. This is used in research designs where each subject acts as his or her own control.

Factorial ANOVA is a combination of two-way and repeated measures ANOVA. It is used to compare the means of two or more groups under two or more conditions at 2 or more points in time, using a single dependent (outcome) variable.

Multivariate analysis of variance (MANOVA) is capable of comparing the means of two or more groups using two or more continuous dependent (outcome) measures.

Analysis of covariance (ANCOVA or MANCOVA) is a variation of ANOVA/ MANOVA in which one or more variables (covariates) are controlled (held constant) to eliminate their biasing effect on the result.

Assumptions of ANOVA

1. In an experiment, participants are randomly allocated to groups.
2. The dependent variable is continuous, measured on an interval scale, and approximates to the normal distribution.
3. The standard deviations for each group or comparison condition are approximately equal (homogeneity of variance).

An important task for the reviewer is to check the descriptive statistics to ensure that the assumptions of normality and homogeneity of variance have been adhered to (see Chapter 4).

Principles of ANOVA

In Chapter 11, we described one-way ANOVA as an extension of the unrelated *t* test. Two-way ANOVA may be regarded as a combination of the related and the unrelated *t* test. It is based on a comparison of group means, taking account of within-group variation (i.e. the standard deviations). For example, a set of results might identify:

- main effect for groups: a measure of the mean differences between the groups at the same point in time;
- main effects for change: a measure of within-group change, based on repeated measures;
- interaction between groups and change.

Claesson et al. (2007) set out to compare weight change over time in two groups of pregnant women recruited from different localities: group A received a weight control programme; group B acted as a control. The dependent variable was weight. The women were weighed at baseline and again following birth. An extract from the data is given in Table 14.2.

Table 14.2 Pre–post intervention weight comparisons (from Claesson et al. 2007)

	Group A ($n = 150$) Intervention group: mean (sd)	Group B ($n = 163$) Control group: mean (sd)
Time 1: Mean weight at 1st antenatal visit (baseline)	95.5 (12.65) kg	95.9 (15.4) kg
Time 2: Mean weight at postnatal check	93.2 (13.32) kg	96.5 (14.48) kg

Both groups weighed about the same at baseline. By follow-up, the intervention group had lost weight and the control group had gained weight. But is this change statistically significant?

ANOVA is the test of choice, but since the women were not randomly allocated to groups, it is important to check for baseline differences. The standard deviations at baseline appear different, so it is necessary to question if the assumption of homogeneity of variance is fulfilled. In this case, the researchers report Levene's test for equality of variance which confirmed no significant difference between groups at baseline.

The result of ANOVA gives three separate values of F, each with its own value of p:

• Main effect for the weight control programme, indicated by between-group differences at follow-up.

• Main effect for change: within groups weight change over time.

• Group × change interaction: if each group responds differently over time, this is shown on a graph by a divergence or crossing of the lines connecting the pre- and post-test values.

It is easier for the reviewer to understand these effects by constructing a graph, as we have done in Figure 14.1. The graph clearly demonstrates that, between baseline and follow-up, the intervention group lost weight while the control group gained weight.

How can we be sure that these results are a consequence of the weight control programme and not some other factor related, for example, to different demographics? Claesson et al. used ANCOVA to control for differences in age, parity, socio-economic status, occupation and smoking. The result of ANCOVA confirmed the significant impact of the weight control programme.

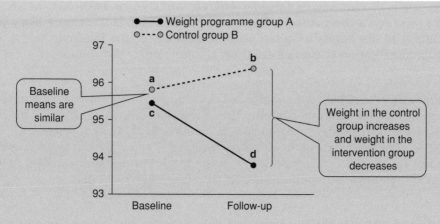

Figure 14.1 Graph of weight change, based on data from Table 14.2 (Claesson et al. 2007)

As with one-way ANOVA and ANCOVA, post-hoc multiple comparison tests are required to locate the precise source of difference (see Chapter 12 and the example in Chapter 1).

What particular problems should the reviewer look out for?

Factorial ANOVA and ANCOVA are based on complex research designs and require large sample sizes. The reviewer should look to see if the sample size was based on power calculations.

- If no sample size calculation was done, the study may be underpowered, which might lead to Type II error (failure to classify a result as significant when it really is).
- If it was based on a power calculation, the reviewer should look at the degrees of freedom recorded in the results to ensure that the number of observations included in the analysis has not fallen below this figure due to attrition or missing data.
- Check that the data for each group at each point in time approximates to the normal distribution (see Chapter 4 for guidance on what to look for).
- Check that the standard deviations for groups are comparable (this is the assumption of homogeneity of variance). If they appear different, look to see if the researchers conducted Levene's test for equality of variance. A non-significant result on this test ($p > 0.05$) indicates no differences in the group variances.

Friedman two-way analysis of variance by ranks

Although presented as the equivalent of two-way ANOVA, this is actually an extension of the Wilcoxon signed rank test (see Chapter 13) and is the nonparametric equivalent of the repeated measures ANOVA. There is no nonparametric equivalent of two-way or factorial ANOVA, ANCOVA or MANOVA, which is why most researchers strive to use a continuous dependent measure likely to conform to the normal distribution. The main use of the Friedman test is in longitudinal cohort studies where there are non-normal distributions.

Example

Johansson et al. (2008) were interested in finding out how fatigue varied over time in multiple sclerosis patients. They measured fatigue using the Fatigue Severity Scale (FSS) and collected data at baseline, 6, 12, 18 and 24 months.

The researchers state in their Analysis section that the Friedman test was used to test for changes in FSS scores. In reporting the results, the researchers state that FSS scores varied significantly over time ($p = 0.02$, $n = 197$).

As with ANOVA, the Friedman test only indicates that *at least one of* the conditions differs from *at least one of* the other conditions. Post-hoc comparisons are conducted using a series of paired Wilcoxon signed rank tests. The level of probability should be lowered to reduce the likelihood of Type I error (see Bonferroni correction in Chapter 8).

Cochrane Q test

This is an extension of McNemar's test (Chapter 13) where the dependent measure is dichotomous (success or failure) and repeated measures are taken at three or more points in time. The value of Q (the test statistic) is interpreted using the tables for χ^2 with $k - 1$ degrees of freedom (where there are k conditions or measurement points).

Summary

The following tests may be used to compare multiple groups and/or repeated measurements:

- two-way or factorial ANOVA, a parametric test, if the dependent measure is continuous and approximates to the normal distribution, and the group distributions are statistically comparable (homogeneity of variance);

- Friedman two-way ANOVA by ranks, a nonparametric test to compare repeated measurements over multiple time points, if the dependent measure is ordinal or the assumptions for ANOVA cannot be met;

- Cochrane Q test, if the dependent measure consists of frequency counts in mutually exclusive, unrelated categories.

15 Simple Tests of Association: Correlation and Linear Regression

KEY QUESTIONS

- What is a correlation?
- What is the difference between correlation and regression?
- How do I interpret correlation?
- What should I look for in the results?

Introduction

This chapter focuses on simple statistical tests to measure the strength of relationship between two variables.

Correlation is used to test the strength of the relationship between a paired set of measurements. Correlation does not imply causation.

Regression is very similar to correlation but is based on the assumption that there is a causal relationship between one or more predictor (independent) variables and one outcome (dependent variable).

Correlation

Correlation measures of the strength of relationship between two variables or measurements, such that as the values on one measurement change, values on the other measurement also change.

Correlation is only possible if the two sets of measurements are paired, as in:

- two different sets of measurements taken from the same sample of individuals;
- the same set of measurements taken from matched pairs of individuals;
- the same set of measurements taken from the same sample of individuals at two different points in time.

The relationship must be linear (approximate to a straight line), as opposed to curvilinear (follow a curved line).

Assuming that the variables are continuous or ordinal, correlation is best understood using a 'scatterplot' in which the data for one variable are plotted against the data for the other, as illustrated in Figure 15.1. The closer the plotted values to the line of best fit, the higher the level of correlation. Tests of correlation may be parametric and nonparametric.

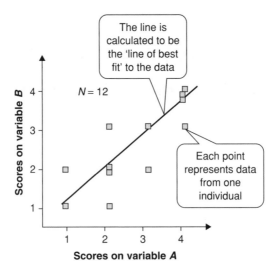

Figure 15.1 Illustration of scatterplot of data taken from within the same sample

Parametric tests of correlation

The **Pearson product-moment correlation**, recognised by the correlation coefficient, r, is usually used if both variables are measured using a continuous scale and the data are spread across the full range of values.

Partial correlation is a version of Pearson correlation which is used to measure the association between two variables while using statistical control to eliminate the effect of a third confounding variable.

Nonparametric tests of correlation

Nonparametric tests include **Spearman's rho** (r_s) and **Kendall's tau** (τ).

• These tests are used if either variable is measured using an ordinal scale or a continuous measurement that has a skewed or unusual distribution. They are both rank-order tests (see Chapter 5 for an explanation of rank measurements).

• Spearman is the most powerful and commonly used nonparametric test of correlation.

• Kendall's tau is used for odd distributions and has the advantage of being able to deal with partial correlation.

Phi (Φ or r_Φ) is used where both variables are dichotomous (a characteristic that is either present or absent). Correlation cannot be used for other forms of categorical data.

Interpretation of the correlation coefficient

Although calculated differently, all correlation coefficients produce a number between −1 and +1.

- 0 represents no association between the two variables.
- ±1 represents a perfect association between the two variables.
- A positive correlation means that as scores on one variable increase, scores on the other also increase.
- A negative correlation coefficient (indicated by a minus sign) means that as scores on one variable increase, scores on the other decrease.

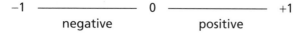

Positive and negative correlations are illustrated in Figure 15.2.

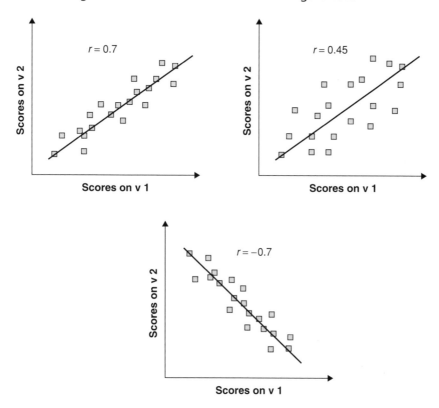

Figure 15.2 Scatterplots showing positive and negative correlations

The interpretation of the correlation coefficient is more stringent in the natural sciences, including medical science, where measurements are very precise, compared to the social sciences where measurements are less precise. We have indicated our interpretation in Figure 15.3.

Natural sciences

0.8–1   Strong relationship
0.6–0.79   Moderate relationship
0.4–0.59   Weak relationship

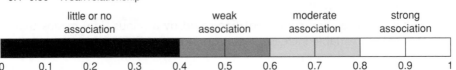

Social sciences

0.6–1   Strong relationship
0.3–0.59   Moderate to fairly strong relationship
0.15–0.3   Weak relationship

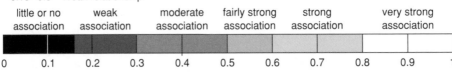

Figure 15.3 Rough guide to interpreting correlation coefficients in the natural and social sciences

Kovacs et al. (2004) used correlations to establish the relationship between pain and disability, between pain and quality of life, and between disability and quality of life. Findings from different points in time included:

- Pain × disability (day 1), $r = 0.347$: moderate relationship – as pain increases, disability increases.
- Pain × quality of life (day 15), $r = -0.672$: strong relationship – as pain increases, quality of life decreases.
- Disability × quality of life (day 1), $r = -0.442$: moderate relationship – as disability increases, quality of life decreases.

The meaning of correlation

The reviewer must ask three questions:

1. What is the direction of the relationship? You may need to look at the scoring to see if high scores imply a negative or a positive state.
2. Does the correlation coefficient indicate a strong, moderate or weak relationship? A significant correlation may nevertheless be weak.
3. Is the relationship statistically significant? If not, the result is not meaningful.

In the Kovacs et al. (2004) study, the relationship for pain × disability was: $r = 0.347$, $n = 195$, $p = 0.000$.

$r = 0.347$ means that there is a moderate, positive correlation between pain and disability.

$n = 195$ means that 195 patients returned a complete set of data for both variables.

$p = 0.000$ indicates that the likelihood that there is *no* relationship is less than 1:1000. This suggests the relationship is strongly statistically significant.

The researchers do not state if a one-tailed or two-tailed test of probability was used (see Chapter 9 for the importance of this), so the reviewer might want to check this using statistical tables, see Table 15.1.

Table 15.1 Extract from statistical table for Pearson correlation coefficient, showing interpretation of $r = 0.347$ if $n \geq 100$

n (Sample size)	Directional (one tailed) p				
	0.05	0.025	0.01	0.005	0.0005
	Non-directional (two tailed) p				
	0.1	0.05	0.025	0.01	0.001
20	0.36	0.42	0.49	0.54	0.65
30	0.30	0.35	0.45	0.51	0.55
50	0.23	0.27	0.32	0.35	0.44
100	0.16	0.19	0.23	0.25	0.32

If $r = 0.347$ (moderate), $n > 100$
one-tailed $p < 0.0005$
two-tailed $p < 0.001$

Look along the bottom row in Table 15.1 at values of r where the sample size is 100+. A value of $r \geq 0.32$ achieves $p < 0.001$ if a two-tailed test of probability is applied, and $p < 0.000$ if a one-tailed test is used (it is usual to give significance to no more than 3 decimal places). It would appear that Kovacs used a one-tailed test of probability.

Now assume that the number of complete data sets returned was only 30. Look along the row for $n = 30$ in Table 15.1 and you will see that a correlation coefficient of $r = 0.347$ achieves $p < 0.05$ (statistically significant) if a one-tailed test of probability was applied, but a p value between 0.1 and 0.05 (not significant) if a two-tailed test of probability was applied.

Note that:

- A weak correlation will achieve statistical significance if the sample size is sufficiently large.
- A moderate correlation will not achieve statistical significance if the sample size is too small.

Presentation of correlation findings

Correlation results may be presented in the form of text, table or correlation matrix. Results often appear in the following types of format:

- Increase in pain was associated with an increase in disability ($r = 0.347$, $n = 195$; two-tailed $p < 0.001$).
- As predicted, the more pain people reported, the greater their level of disability ($r(195) = 0.347$, $p < 0.000$).

In either case r gives the strength of the relationship on the scale of 0 to 1; p indicates the statistical significance of the association; and n indicates the number of cases (respondents) included in the analysis. It is worth checking the value of n against the original sample size to check the extent of missing data.

If several variables are compared, a correlation matrix is an efficient way of presenting the results. The value of p may be included in the table (as in Kovacs et al. 2004) or indicated using a star system, as in Table 15.2.

Table 15.2 Correlation matrix showing relationship between pain, quality of life and disability (from Kovacs et al. 2004)

	Pain	Disability
Disability	0.347* ($n = 195$)	
Quality of life	0.672* ($n = 164$, day 15)	0.442* ($n = 195$)

*$p < 0.001$

Correlation does not imply causation

Just because the change in one variable *is associated with* a change in the other, that does *not* imply that one *causes* the other. Consider possible relationships between disability and quality of life in the Kovacs et al. example:

- Disability causes a decrease in quality of life.
- A decrease in quality of life, caused by social problems, leads to an increase in pain behaviours and disability.
- Pain causes both an increase in disability and a decrease in quality of life.
- Measures of disability and quality of life share similar items on the measurement scales, so that they are partly measuring the same thing.

The reviewer must consider alternative explanations and be convinced that the researchers are fully justified in their interpretation of the findings.

Curvilinear relationships

Some relationships follow a curved line, rather than a straight line, as indicated in Figure 15.4. Correlation usually shows no relationship, though this is misleading.

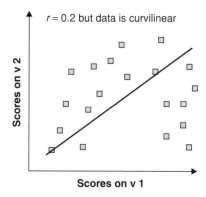

Figure 15.4 Scatterplot showing a curvilinear relationship

Curved-line relationships, such as the one illustrated, are a fairly common feature of the relationship between psychological and physiological measurements, for example the relationship between physiological arousal and cognitive performance (the Yerkes–Dodson law). The reviewer must rely on the researchers to report on their inspection of scatterplots of their data.

If a relationship is curvilinear, you may see that the researchers report having 'transformed' the data. This involves using a mathematical device such as logarithm or square root in order to achieve a linear relationship.

Partial correlation

Partial correlation enables the researcher to establish a correlation between two variables, while controlling for (eliminating) the effect of a third confounding variable. This is similar to the concept of the covariate in analysis of covariance (ANCOVA; see Chapter 14).

For example, it would be possible to establish the relationship between disability and quality of life while controlling for the level of pain. This would reveal the 'true' relationship between disability and quality of life without the confounding effects of pain.

Regression analysis

The main difference between correlation and regression is that, whereas correlation does not imply causation, regression does. Regression should only be used when the researchers justify a theoretical relationship between one or more independent (predictor) variables and one dependent (outcome) variable.

The result of regression analysis includes a regression equation which takes the form of a straight-line equation. This means that if an individual's score on one or more predictor variables is known, their score (or risk) on the outcome variable can be calculated. Therefore, regression analysis is well suited to use in epidemiological research.

The main forms of regression analysis are:

- **simple linear regression**, which has one continuous predictor variable and one continuous outcome (dependent) variable;
- **multiple regression**, which includes more than one continuous or dichotomous predictor variable and one continuous outcome variable;
- **logistic regression**, which includes more than one predictor variable, which may be continuous or categorical, and one dichotomous outcome variable.

Simple linear regression

Simple linear regression predicts the relationship between one independent variable X (the cause) and one dependent variable Y (the effect). The variables X and Y must both be continuous and must approximate to the normal distribution. The results of simple linear regression include:

- the regression coefficient R;
- the regression equation that specifies the numerical value of Y for each value of X.

The regression coefficient R

The regression coefficient R is interpreted in the same way as the correlation coefficient r on a scale of 0 to 1. But this actually inflates the ability of the independent variable to predict the value of the dependent variable. We use R^2 (the square of R) as a measure of the proportion of 'shared variance' between the two variables, which gives a much more realistic idea of the strength of the causal relationship.

The value of R^2 is usually given as a percentage, rather than as a decimal. If the researchers fail to give the R^2 value, it is easy to work it out; see Table 15.3.

Table 15.3 Conversion of R values to R^2

R	R^2
0.9	0.81 (81%)
0.8	0.64 (64%)
0.7	0.49 (49%)
0.6	0.36 (36%)
0.5	0.25 (25%)
0.4	0.16 (16%)
0.3	0.09 (9%)
0.2	0.04 (4%)

The regression equation (regression model)

The regression equation is the equation for a straight line:

$Y = A + BX$.

These symbols have the following meanings:

Y is the individual's score on the dependent variable.

X is the individual's score on the predictor (independent) variable.

B is the weighting given to the independent variable.

A is a constant which gives the value of Y when $X = 0$.

This relationship is illustrated in Figure 15.5, using imaginary data.

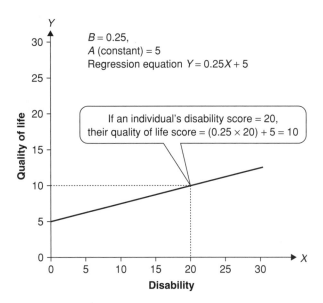

Figure 15.5 Graph of the regression line showing imaginary relationship between disability and quality of life

Assumptions of simple linear regression

1. The researcher must present a plausible theoretical explanation for a causal relationship between the predictor and outcome variable.

2. Both variables must be measured using a continuous, interval scale.

3. The distribution of both variables should approximate to the normal distribution or be fairly evenly distributed across the range of values.

4. The relationship between the independent and dependent variables must follow a straight line.

Real life is really too complex to focus on a simple causal relationship between two variables. Health and social researchers usually collect measurements relating to a number of possible predictor variables and analyse their joint impact, using multiple regression. We cover this in the next chapter.

Summary

- Correlation tests the strength, direction and significance of relationship between two variables taken from two independent groups, or from the same group on two separate occasions.
- Simple linear regression predicts the strength, direction and mathematical formula for the causal relationship between two variables, based on a straight-line equation.

16 Complex Associations:
Multiple and Logistic Regression

KEY QUESTIONS

- What is the purpose of these tests?
- What assumptions need to be met for the results of these tests to be valid?
- How should I interpret the results of these tests?
- What is meant by odds ratio, relative risk and number needed to treat?

Multiple regression

Multiple regression is based on the same principle as simple linear regression, but is used to establish the relationship between several continuous or dichotomous independent variables (predictors or risk factors) and one continuous dependent (outcome) variable.

Multiple regression is popular in epidemiological research because the resulting regression equation enables clinicians to predict an individual's likely health outcome from their scores on one or more independent risk factors.

Multiple regression is based on the assumption that there is a cause and effect relationship between a set of predictor variables (risk factors) and the dependent (outcome) variable. Therefore the analysis is only valid if there is sound theoretical or research-based justification for entering each predictor variable into the regression analysis.

The regression model

The purpose of multiple regression analysis is to select the best combination of independent (predictor) variables (X_1, X_2, etc.) that predict the value of the dependent (outcome) variable (Y). This is known as the regression model because it reflects a theoretical model of cause and effect. The regression model is illustrated in Figure 16.1.

The regression model is determined by the following criteria:

- Each predictor must make a statistically significant contribution to the prediction of the dependent variable. This is tested using individual t tests.

- The combination of predictors must explain a statistically significant proportion of the variance associated with the dependent variable. This is tested using analysis of variance (the F test), which should be statistically significant.

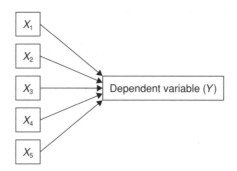

Figure 16.1 Regression model

The regression model is described in mathematical terms by the regression equation, which is a straight-line equation:

$Y = B_1X_1 + B_2X_2 + \ldots + A.$

In this equation:

Y is the value of the dependent (outcome) variable.

X_1, X_2, etc. represent each independent (predictor) variables.

B_1, B_2, etc. are the weightings given to each independent variable by the regression equation.

A is a constant that reflects the value of Y when all values of $X = 0$.

Example

Recall the *imaginary* example of children fidgeting that we referred to in Chapters 11 and 13. From a list of predictors entered into the regression analysis, three (sex, age and parental control score) are selected into the regression model as the best predictors of fidgeting (measured by minutes of focused attention during a 10-minute period of observation). The result of multiple regression analysis gives the regression equation as:

minutes of focused attention = 3.01 × male sex + 0.52 × age + 0.6 × score on parental control + 15.

Thus (in theory) it would be possible to predict the attention span for each individual child provided their sex, age and score on parental control are known.

Assumptions of multiple regression

Multiple regression is conceptually simple, but is based on quite a lot of assumptions:

1. The regression model is one of cause and effect. Therefore, the researcher should present a plausible theoretical explanation for the causal relationship between each predictor and the dependent variable.

2. The dependent variable is a continuous measure that approximates to the normal distribution.

3. The predictors must be measured using either a continuous, interval scale that approximates to the normal distribution, or a dichotomous measure (a characteristic that is either present or absent). There are arguments for including ordinal variables such as those measured using a five-point Likert scale of response, but the analysis cannot cope with categorical data (other than dichotomous variables).

4. The relationship between each predictor and the dependent variable must be linear. Where curvilinear relationships exist (see Chapter 15), the researchers may 'transform' the data using square roots or logarithms to achieve linearity.

5. There must *not* be a strong correlation between any pair of independent variables. A high correlation (be suspicious of anything above 0.7) between pairs of predictors is referred to as 'multicollinearity'. This means that the variables provide similar information, therefore one of them is likely to be excluded from the regression model during analysis (but it might not be the right one). If suspected, multicollinearity may be verified statistically using the **'variance inflation factor' (VIF)**.

6. You may see reference to 'homoscedasticity'. This is a requirement that the predictors and dependent variable have roughly equal standard deviations. Suffice it to say that the researcher should confirm that the assumption of homoscedasticity was met.

The process of regression analysis

It is helpful for a reviewer to have an idea of the procedure in order to understand some of the critical issues involved in this interesting analytical procedure. Figure 16.2 illustrates the analytic stages.

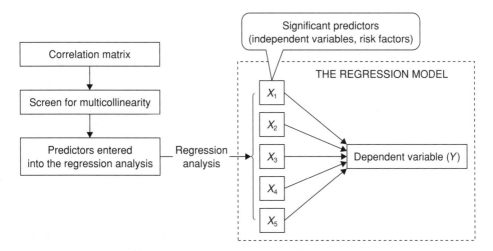

Figure 16.2 Analytic stages in regression analysis

The first step is to produce a correlation matrix that includes each of the predictors and the dependent variable. This serves two purposes, which the reviewer can check:

- Predictors that do not show a significant correlation with the dependent variable are excluded from the regression analysis.
- A high correlation (usually above 0.8) between a pair of predictors suggests collinearity and requires investigation.

The screened predictors are then entered into the regression analysis one at a time, usually starting with the one that shows the highest correlation with the dependent variable (Y).

Each time a predictor is entered, the predictive contribution of those already in the regression model is held constant. This means that if there is a correlation between two or more predictors in the regression model, the first ones entered take up all of the variance they share with the dependent variable. Therefore, unless the predictors are entirely independent of each other, the order of entry can make a big difference to the final regression model.

There are several methods of entering predictor variables into the regression analysis. As a reviewer, you are most likely to encounter the following:

- Forward selection in an order determined by the researcher, usually on theoretical grounds.
- Backward elimination to check if the order changes as each predictor is removed from the model.
- Stepwise selection in which the computer starts by including the predictor that shows the strongest correlation with the dependent variable. Then each predictor is included according to the strength of its residual correlation until no further predictors make a significant contribution to the regression model.

Example

Table 16.1 Table of regression results, based on the fidget study

Dependent variable: Minutes of focused attention during 1 hour of observation ($n = 64$)				
Independent variable	B	β	t	p
Sex (male)	3.01	0.5	3.4	0.001
Age	0.52	0.3	2.6	0.01
Parental control	0.6	0.03	1.6	ns
Constant	15.0		3.5	0.001

Adjusted $R^2 = 0.23$.

R^2 = proportion of variance in the data explained by the regression model

B = weighting of each independent variable in the regression model

β = Relative importance of each independent variable

t test of significance for each independent variable

Interpreting the results of multiple regression

The results of multiple regression are usually given in the form of a table. Table 16.1 uses the example from our imaginary study of fidgeting to illustrate key information contained within a typical table of results.

- Values of B give the weighting of each independent variable in the regression equation. In Table 16.1, minutes of focused attention for an individual child is predicted by:

  (3.01, if male) + (0.52 × age) + (0.6 × parental control) + 15
- Values of β give the relative importance of each variable in relation to each other.
- The significance of each variable within the regression model is tested using a t test and indicated by the value of p (in Table 16.1, parental control is not significant and should actually be excluded)
- The value of R^2 gives the total amount of variation explained by the combination of independent variables in the regression model. It is often given as a percentage (i.e. 0.23 = 23%).
- The overall fit of the regression model in explaining the dependent variable is tested using ANOVA, which should give a significant value of F.

Examples 1 and 2 illustrate different approaches to analysis and presentation.

A large-scale study by Torgerson et al. (1995) sought to identify predictors of bone mass density in women aged 40–49. The results are given in Table 16.2.

Example 1

Table 16.2 Results of regression analysis (from Torgerson et al. 1995)

Independent variables normally given in the order they are entered into the regression equation

Dependent variable: bone mass density in the greater trochanter			
Independent variable	Coefficient (B)	95% CI (B)	Significance (p)
Current weight (kg)	0.0049	0.0044, 0.0054	<0.0001
Exercise per week (hours)	−0.0087	−0.0127, −0.0046	<0.0001
Mother smoked	−0.0201	−0.0321, −0.0080	0.0011
History of wrist fracture	−0.0344	−0.567, −0.0121	0.0025
(constant)	0.4407	0.4068, 0.4746	<0.0001

Adjusted R^2 = 26.0%

This combination of independent variables explains 26% of the variance associated with bone mass density

These values give the regression equation. They have no meaning in relation to each other

CI and p confirm that each independent variable makes a significant contribution to the regression model

Results in the column marked **coefficient B** indicate that increased weight has a positive impact on bone density. Minus signs indicate that the other factors have a negative effect on bone density. The actual values and confidence intervals for B cannot be directly compared because they relate to different units of measurement.

Reading down the column labelled coefficient B, the values of B give the regression equation as:

bone density = (0.0049 × weight) − (0.0087 × hours of exercise) − 0.0201 × mother was smoker) − (0.0344 × history of wrist fracture) + 0.4407.

Confidence intervals (CI) for B do not straddle 0, indicating that each predictor makes a statistically significant contribution to the regression model. These indicate the range of weightings that would need to be taken into account when making clinical predictions. Values of p are all statistically significant ($p < 0.05$).

The R^2 **value** indicates that the independent variables combine to explain 26% of the variance associated with bone density in this group of women.

Clearly, there are other factors operating to predict bone density, but this study makes an important contribution to preventive medicine.

Example 2

Table 16.3 Table of regression results (from Keeley et al. 2008)

Dependent variable: Physical quality of life (disability) 6 months following baseline			
Independent variables		β	p
Block 1	(constant)		<0.0005
	Age	−0.048	0.61
	Education	−0.02	0.83
Block 2	Cause of pain	−0.02	0.79
	Duration of pain (years)	−0.18	0.04
Block 3	HADs total score	−0.27	0.003
	FAB activity score	−0.09	0.3
	FAB work score	−0.06	0.55
	Pain-related social stresses	−0.42	<0.0005
	Unrelated social stresses	0.065	0.41

Adjusted $R^2 = 0.5$; $F = 11.2$, $p < 0.0005$.
HADs is the Hospital Anxiety and Depression scale.
FAB is a measure of fear-avoidance behaviour.

Look at the relationship between each relative weighting and significance

Blocks include variables that do not make a significant contribution to the prediction of quality of life

Keeley et al. (2008) sought to predict physical quality of life (disability) after 6 months of treatment for chronic pain, using three 'blocks' of variables representing demographic, pain-related, and psychosocial factors. Demographic variables demonstrating multicollinearity were identified using the variance inflation factor and excluded from the analysis. A total of nine variables were entered into the regression equation in a fixed order (see Table 16.3).

In the table of results, only the p values circled indicate a variable that makes a significant contribution to the regression model. The other variables are all non-significant and have a beta (β) weighting (relative importance) close to zero.

In the Keeley et al. study, the combined power of the independent variables to explain physical quality of life is 50% ($R^2 = 0.5$), and the F test shows that this model is statistically significant. This result appears impressive. However, look closely at them.

- Many of the standardised weightings (β) are close to zero.
- Many of the probability levels (p) do not achieve significance. No demographic variables achieve significance.

Only 'duration of pain', 'HAD score' and 'pain-related social stresses' were significant predictors in the regression model, the most important being pain-related social stress ($\beta = 0.42$, $p < 0.0005$). The inclusion of so many non-significant variables seems likely to have inflated the value of R^2 and overestimated the importance of this regression model.

An additional criticism is that it is not clear how many complete sets of data were included in this analysis. The authors state that 120 people were recruited, of whom 108 completed baseline measures. However, data from a separate table indicate that a maximum of 93 people completed the dependent measure. Did all of these submit complete data for every independent variable? Given the complexity of the analysis, the sample size is small and the study appears underpowered for this type of analysis (see guidance in Chapter 8 on sample size).

Checklist of things to look for in regression results

- Is a cause–effect relationship between each independent variable and the dependent variable predicted by the researchers in their introductory section?
- Is the outcome measure continuous (see Chapter 4) and does it conform to the normal distribution?
- Compare the value of n (complete sets of data in the analysis) with the calculated and actual sample size. Is there much evidence of missing data? Is n large enough (see Chapter 8) for this analysis?
- Check the interrelationship between the independent variables in the correlation matrix (see Chapter 15). Is there any evidence of collinearity? If so, have the researchers addressed this?

- Check the order of entry of the predictors. Is there any evidence that inter-relationship between these might have affected the result?
- Are the values for *B* given? If so, construct the regression equation. Are confidence intervals for *B* given?
- Are the values for beta (β, comparative weightings) given? If so, what is the relative importance for the predictor variables?
- Do each of the independent variables make a significant contribution to the regression model ($p \leq 0.05$)?
- What percentage of the variance (value of R^2) does the regression model account for? What might account for unexplained variance?
- If given, what are the value and significance of *F*? Is the regression a good fit with the data?

Logistic regression

Logistic regression is used to predict a categorical dependent (outcome) variable using two or more categorical or continuous independent (predictor) variables. The dependent variable is usually dichotomous.[1]

Logistic regression is commonly used in public health to predict risk factors for a disease or condition that is either present or absent.

Logistic regression is a 'multidimensional' version of contingency analysis where there can be many predictors and one categorical (usually dichotomous) dependent variable. It has few assumptions in terms of type or distribution of data, but requires a large sample size and is really best suited to large-scale, well-funded studies. The researchers must explain how they arrived at their sample size calculation, making sufficient allowance for missing data.

The conceptual basis of logistic regression is illustrated in Figure 16.3. As with multiple regression, each independent variable is entered in turn into a complex multidimensional computational model. This enables the researchers to identify the effect of each predictor on the dependent variable, while controlling for the other predictors.

The predictors included in the final model are selected because each makes an independent statistically significant contribution to the model. Also, in combination, they form the strongest regression model.

The final statistic, **chi-square (χ^2)**, is used to assess the fit of the final regression model to the data (it is referred to as a test of 'goodness of fit'). In this case, a non-significant test result ($p > 0.05$) is desirable since this indicates that there is *no* significant difference between the regression model and the data – i.e. the model is a 'good fit' with the data.

The effect of each selected predictor on the outcome variable is given as an odds ratio (OR).

---

1 While it is possible to predict a categorical dependent variable, the analysis is complex and logistic regression is usually based on a dichotomous dependent variable.

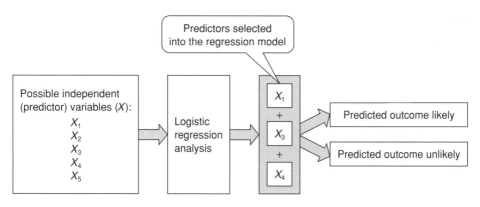

Figure 16.3 Illustration of the process of logistic regression analysis

Thurston et al. (2007) used logistic regression to predict the likelihood that women with higher levels of body fat would report menopausal vasomotor symptoms (hot flushes, night sweats). The dependent variable was the presence or absence of vasomotor symptoms.

The researchers collected complete sets of data from 1,776 women. The data included a range of predictors thought to influence hot flushes. From these, preliminary tests of group difference identified a list of predictors that distinguished between those with and those without vasomotor symptoms. These were then included in the logistic regression analysis (Table 16.4).

Table 16.4 Predictors of hot flushes (from Thurston et al. 2007)

	Significance (*p*)
1. Study site (6 sites)	<0.0001
2. Race/ethnicity (4 groups)	<0.0001
3. Education (college vs less than college educated)	<0.0001
4. Smoker	0.0001
5. Parity (0 or ≥1)	0.012
6. Menopausal stage (pre, early, post)	<0.0001
7. Waist circumference (controlled for % body fat)	<0.0001
8. Anxiety symptoms	<0.0001
9. Follicle-stimulating hormone (FSH) level	<0.0001
10. Estradiol level	<0.0001
11. Free estradiol index (FEI)	<0.0001
12. % body fat	<0.0001

Several variables were entered into the regression analysis first to control for (eliminate) their effects. These 'covariates' were age, site, race/ethnicity, educational attainment, parity, cycle day of blood drawing, smoking status, hormone use in the past month, and anxiety symptoms.

The results of logistic regression showed that percentage of body fat was a significant predictor of hot flushes after 'fully adjusting' for all of the covariates and after controlling for each of the hormonal factors in turn. The results are given as odds ratios (OR), a measure of effect size, as illustrated in Table 16.5.

Table 16.5 Table of results of logistic regression, giving odds ratios (from Thurston et al. 2007)

95% confidence interval gives range of values predicted with certainty if $\alpha = 0.05$

	Fully adjusted + FSH		Fully adjusted + estradiol		Fully adjusted + FEI	
	OR	95% CI	OR	95% CI	OR	95% CI
% body fat	1.19**	1.05, 1.34	1.15*	1.01, 1.29	1.20**	1.06, 1.36

$*p < 0.05$; $**p < 0.01$.
FSH Follicle Stimulating Hormone; FEI Free Estradiol Index.

The results demonstrated that increased body fat leads to reports of hot flushes in perimenopausal women. This relationship persisted even after controlling for a range of other influences, including waist circumference and hormone levels.

Odds ratio (OR)

Unlike multiple regression, the results of logistic regression are usually given as a series of odds ratios which measure the impact of each predictor (or risk factor) on the dependent variable (the outcome).

The odds ratio (OR) refers to the odds of being in one category, compared to the odds of being in the alternative category. Take the example in Table 16.6. Here the proportion of people with *high* body fat who get hot flushes is a/b, and the proportion of people with *low* body fat who get hot flushes is c/d. The odds ratio is the ratio of these two proportions:

$$OR = \frac{a/b}{c/d}.$$

Table 16.6 Body fat and hot flushes

	Hot flushes present	Hot flushes absent
High proportion of body fat	a	b
Low proportion of body fat	c	d

An odds ratio of 1 indicates that the odds of being in either category are the same. Using the example of body fat as a predictor of hot flushes:

- OR = 1 would indicate that increased body fat was unable to distinguish those reporting hot flushes from those not reporting hot flushes.
- OR > 1 indicates that there is a greater likelihood of having hot flushes, compared to not having hot flushes.
- OR = 1.5 indicates a 50% greater likelihood of having hot flushes, compared to not having hot flushes.
- OR = 2 indicates double the risk of having hot flushes, compared to the likelihood of not having hot flushes.

The OR must be significant ($p < 0.05$) to be considered important. This is the same as saying that both values for the 95% confidence interval (CI) must be greater than 1.

In the Thurston study, the mean percentage of body fat was 37.9 (standard deviation = 7.8). Their findings indicate that an increase of one standard deviation in percentage of body fat had a significant effect on hot flushes, even after controlling for a variety of other significant influences including hormonal effects.

How big was this effect? Taking account of the confidence intervals, the effect size ranged from a minimum of 1.01 (virtually no effect) to a maximum of 1.36.

An OR of 1.36 indicates a 36% increase in likelihood of having hot flushes (compared to the likelihood of not having hot flushes) for each additional standard deviation increase in percentage of body fat.

Example

We give a detailed worked example of the odds ratio in Chapter 1.

Relative risk (RR)

Relative risk or benefit (RR) is an alternative to the odds ratio. Whereas OR is commonly used in RCTs, RR is more commonly used in epidemiology.

It refers to the proportion in one group or condition that experienced a negative or positive outcome, compared to the proportion in the other group or condition that experienced a negative or positive outcome. Using the data in Table 16.6, the relative risk of developing hot flushes due to a high proportion of body fat is given by

$$RR = \frac{a/(a+b)}{c/(c+d)}.$$

We give a worked example of this in Chapter 1, where we contrast it with odds ratio.

Note that it is essential that values for OR and RR should never be regarded as precise for clinical purposes. They must be accompanied by confidence intervals that give the range of values likely to be found in the population 95% or 99% of the time, depending on the level of probability set (see Chapter 9).

Number needed to treat (NNT)

The number needed to treat (NNT) is an important outcome measure used in clinical trials. It is the number of people who need to receive an intervention in order for one to achieve clinical benefit (see the example in Chapter 1). It is also used to predict adverse events, in which case it is interpreted as the number needed to harm.

Take the example of Table 16.6. NNT is the number needed to be treated in a weight control programme to reduce the proportion of body fat, in order for one person to cease having hot flushes. To calculate this we proceed as follows.

- Calculate the proportion of people with *high* body fat who have hot flushes: $a/(a + b)$.
- Calculate the proportion of people with *low* body fat who have hot flushes: $c/(c + d)$.
- Take the difference between these two proportions, and take its reciprocal (which just means divide 1 by it).

We write this in symbols as

$$NNT = \frac{1}{\left(\frac{a}{a+b}\right) - \left(\frac{c}{c+d}\right)}.$$

Clearly, a weight control programme to reduce body fat from high to low would be very ambitious. Therefore, a more sensible approach is to do like Thurston et al. and calculate the NNT in order to reduce weight by one standard deviation.

As with OR and RR, the confidence interval for NNT is essential when determining the clinical impact of an intervention.

Summary

- Multiple regression predicts the strength, direction and mathematical formula for the causal relationships between one or more dichotomous or continuous predictor variables (risk factors) and one outcome variable. It is used if certain parametric assumptions are met.
- Logistic regression is used where the dependent variable is dichotomous and the results given in odds ratio form.

Further reading

Bandolier (2008) *Effect size.* http://www.medicine.ox.ac.uk/bandolier/booth/glossary/effect.html (accessed 19 December 2008).

PART 4
QUICK REFERENCE GUIDE

This section is intended as a reminder and source of immediate information when conducting your own review.

I Framework for Statistical Review

This framework highlights important questions to ask as you read through a research paper. They are presented in a logical sequence, rather than order of priority:

Refer to:

INTRODUCTION

Aim

- What is the main aim or research question?
- What, if any, are the predictions or hypotheses?
- Are predictions stated using the language of certainty or uncertainty?

Background/Introduction

- Do the researchers offer strong evidence in support of their predictions, or is the outcome uncertain?

Chapter 9

METHOD

Sample

- Based on published data and your own experience, does the sample appear representative of the study population and those you encounter in your own practice?

Chapter 6

- Taking account of attrition, missing data and uneven distributions, is the sample size sufficient to support the statistical analyses used?

Chapters 1, 2, 8

- In the case of randomisation to groups, which method was used and was this successful?

Chapters 1, 7

Data measurement

- Have the measures used been properly tested as valid and reliable?
- Are the measures appropriate for use with this study population?

Chapter 6

Planned data analysis

- Do the researchers justify the statistical tests and tests of probability used?

| Chapter 9 and Part 3 |

RESULTS

Descriptive (demographic and baseline) statistics

- Were the descriptive statistics appropriate to the type and distribution of the data?
- If means and standard deviations are used, have the researchers confirmed that the data approximate to the normal distribution?
- Can you spot any clues that continuous data do not conform to the normal distribution?
- Did the researchers provide sufficient information for the reviewer to make an informed judgement about the appropriate application of statistical tests?

| Chapters 3, 4, 5 |

Inferential statistical analysis

- Were the statistical tests used appropriate to the type and distribution of the data?
- Were the assumptions of each statistical test fulfilled?
- If repeated measures were used, were the groups comparable at baseline?
- Did the statistical tests used answer the original research questions?
- Were the significance levels used appropriate to the number of tests used?

| Chapters 4, 5 and Part 3 |
| Part 3 |
| Chapter 9 |

DISCUSSION AND CONCLUSIONS

- Do the researchers take account of all the limitations you have identified?
- Are the conclusions fully justified by the research and its results?

| Chapters 1, 2 |

OUTCOME

- What are the conclusions of your review?

II Glossary of Terms

A priori (before the event) refers to statistical analyses planned in advance to test the main hypotheses.

Alpha (α) has two meanings:

1. Significance level. [Chapter 9]

2. Cronbach's alpha. [Chapter 6]

Analysis of variance (ANOVA) and analysis of covariance (ANCOVA) Tests of group difference. [Chapters 12 and 14]

Attrition refers to avoidable and unavoidable losses from the sample following recruitment. [Chapters 7 and 8]

Bonferroni correction is used to determine the appropriate significance level where multiple tests are carried out on the same set of data. [Chapter 9]

Canonical correlation is used in multivariate tests, such as discriminant function analysis, as a measure of the relationship between a set of independent (predictor) variables and a set of dependent (outcome) variables.

Chi-square analysis (contingency analysis) is a test of group difference used when the dependent (outcome) variable consists of unrelated categories (such as different characteristics or locations). [Chapter 11]

Clinical importance or relevance: in a clinical trial, this refers to a level of improvement judged to be of clinical benefit. A statistically significant outcome may or may not be of clinical importance. [Chapter 9]

Coefficient alpha (Cronbach's alpha or α) is a measure of the internal consistency of a measurement scale. [Chapter 6]

Collinearity implies that two variables are strongly correlated. See also multicollinearity. [Chapter 16]

Communality: a value that indicates the contribution of an individual item to its factor in factor analysis.

Confidence interval (CI) refers to the range of values within which the true value is likely to be found the given percentage of the time (usually 95% or 99%). [Chapter 9]

Contingency analysis – see chi-square analysis.

Contingency table: A simple table used in conjunction with contingency analysis (chi-square analysis). [Chapter 11]

Continuous measurement scale/variable: a measure with equal intervals that normally has at least 11 equidistant points on the scale. [Chapter 3]

Convenience sampling refers to a sample of people who are easily accessible or available. [Chapter 7]

Correlation refers to a statistical test of association used to evaluate the strength of relationship between two interval or ordinal variables. [Chapter 11]

Correlation coefficient (*r*) measures the strength of the relationship between two variables. It is measured on a scale of 0 to 1 where 0 indicates no relationship and 1 (or −1) indicates a perfect relationship. [Chapter 11]

Correlation matrix is a table of all possible paired correlations between several variables. [Chapter 11]

Covariate refers to a potentially confounding variable that is controlled for (held constant) during multivariate statistical analyses such as ANCOVA or multiple regression.

Critical value in a set of statistical tables refers to the minimum value required to achieve significance, given the degrees of freedom and level of probability shown.

Cronbach's alpha – see **coefficient alpha**.

Curvilinear refers to data that follow a curved line when the two variables are plotted against each other on a graph. It is not possible to analyse these data in this form using correlation or regression. [Chapter 11]

Data transformation is used in regression analysis when the relationships between variables are curvilinear (follow a curve, rather than a straight line). Logarithms, square roots or other mathematical devices may be used to eliminate the curve. [Chapter 11]

Degrees of freedom (df): closely related to sample or category size, but with a small reduction to reduce the likelihood of overestimating statistical significance where the sample size is small. [Chapter 10]

Dependent variable refers to the variable that is used to measure the effect of change (the outcome measure). [Chapter 10]

Dichotomous is used to refer to a variable that has only two categories, for example a feature (such as disease) that is either present or absent.

Directional test of probability (one-tailed test): tests the hypothesis that there will be a difference between groups or relationship between variables and the effect can only be in one direction (either positive or negative). [Chapter 9]

Discriminant function analysis is similar to multiple regression, but is used where the dependent variable is ordinal or categorical. The result is judged by the proportion of hits and misses in group classification.

Distribution refers to the pattern of values for a particular variable – see normal distribution and skewed distribution. [Chapter 4]

Effect size is a standardised measure of improvement or change, used to calculate sample size. [Chapter 8]

Generalisability refers to the extent to which the results from the study sample will apply to similar groups in other locations. This is only possible if the sample is truly representative of the population from which it is drawn. [Chapter 7]

Goodness of fit refers to a test that indicates whether or not the results of a statistical test represent a good fit to the data.

Histogram: A graph of interval data, similar to a bar chart but without gaps between each of the bars.

Homogeneity of variance means that the variances or standard deviations of the dependent (outcome) variable for two or more comparison groups are approximately the same. It is an important assumption for the *t* test and ANOVA or ANCOVA.

Homoscedasticity: An assumption in regression that the degree of variation around the regression line is the same for all values of the predictor variable. Failure of this assumption will affect the reliability of the findings.

Hypothesis: predicts that there will be a difference between two or more groups or a relationship between two or more variables (sometimes referred to as the alternative hypothesis, as opposed to the null hypothesis). [Chapter 9]

Independent variable: A variable that is likely to influence or affect an outcome or change – for example, demographic variables, individual differences or group allocation in a clinical trial. [Chapter 3]

Inferential statistics refers to statistical tests that are used to draw inferences about differences between groups or relationships between variables within a population. [Chapters 10 and 11]

Intention-to-treat analysis is a method of substitution used to compensate for attrition in a clinical trial. [Chapter 7]

Interquartile range: gives the range of measurements for the 50% whose values lie between the 25th and the 75th percentile. [Chapter 6]

Interval data or variable: Data measured using an interval scale. This is a numerical scale of magnitude that has equal intervals between each point on the scale (interval scale). [Chapter 5]

Kendall's tau: an alternative test to Spearman's rho and interpreted in the same way. [Chapter 11]

Kurtosis is a measure that describes how flat or peaked a distribution is. [Chapter 4]

Levene's test for equality of error variance is a test used to ensure that group standard deviations are not significantly different (i.e. it is check for homogeneity of variance). [Chapter 11]

Linear refers to a relationship that follows (approximately) a straight line when the two variables are plotted against each other on a graph or 'scatterplot'. [Chapter 11]

Linear regression is a test of a causal relationship between an independent (predictor) variable and a dependent (outcome) variable, assuming that the data follow a straight line when plotted on a graph or 'scatterplot'. [Chapter 15]

Logistic regression tests the power of several independent variables to predict one dichotomous dependent variable (such as the presence or absence of an event or disease). [Chapter 11]

MANOVA: multivariate analysis of variance. ANOVA that tests for group differences on a number of difference dependent variables. [Chapter 14]

Mean = numerical average. If the data approximate to the normal distribution, the mean will be close to the centre of the bell-shaped distribution curve and about half way between the highest and lowest values in the range. [Chapter 5]

Median: the middle value when the data are placed in rank order of measurement from the lowest to the highest. [Chapter 6]

Mode: the most commonly occurring value in a set of measurements.

Multicollinearity refers to a problem in regression analysis where there is a high correlation between two or more independent variables. [Chapter 11]

Multiple regression is used to establish a causal relationship between more than one independent (predictor) variable and one dependent (outcome) variable. The dependent variable must be measured using an interval scale. [Chapter 16]

Nominal data (categorical data): This refers to discrete categories that are given a number for the purposes of analysis, but these numbers have no meaningful numerical relationship – as when males are coded 1 and females are coded 2. [Chapter 3]

Non-directional test of probability (two-tailed test): This tests the prediction that there may be a difference or relationship within the data. But the prediction is not certain, or it is not possible to predict if the relationship will be positive or negative. [Chapter 9]

Nonparametric refers to statistical tests used to analyse either ordinal data, or interval data that do not conform to the normal distribution. [Chapter 5]

Normal distribution refers to a naturally occurring symmetrical pattern of variation that looks like an inverted bell-shaped curve when interval data are presented on a graph. [Chapter 5]

Null hypothesis states that there will be *no* difference between the groups, or *no* relationship between the variables. [Chapter 9]

Number needed to treat (NNT) is the number of people who need to receive an intervention in order to achieve one successful outcome. [Chapter 11]

Odds ratio (OR) is a measure of relative risk which measures the probability of an occurrence (such as a disease or other adverse event), compared to its non-occurrence. [Chapter 11]

Ordinal data are data measured using an ordinal scale. The scale has numerical values in ascending or descending rank order, but these values do not necessarily have equal intervals (as in verbal rating scales, such as the Likert scale). [Chapter 3]

Orthogonal refers to a total absence of relationship or correlation between variables.

Outliers are extreme values that lie well outside the range of other values in the data set.

Parametric refers to statistical tests used to analyse data that conform to the normal distribution. [Chapter 5]

Partial correlation refers to the correlation between two variables (*A* and *B*), while holding constant (controlling for) the effect of a third variable (*C*). It removes the confounding effects of *C*. [Chapter 11]

Pearson product-moment correlation coefficient (*r*): tests the strength and significance of the relationship between two interval variables. [Chapter 15]

Percentile: the percentage of the population whose scores lie below the value given.

Population refers to everyone who shares a particular characteristic or set of characteristics. [Chapter 7]

Post hoc tests: Literally, tests carried out 'after the event'. It refers to 'pairwise comparisons' carried out between each pair of variables when a significant result has been obtained from analysis of variance (ANOVA or ANCOVA). [Chapter 10]

Power: statistical power refers to the probability that a particular statistical test will detect a statistically significant relationship in the data, assuming that there actually is one. [Chapter 7]

Principle components analysis (PCA): similar to and often used as a preliminary stage in factor analysis to identify which combination of variables explains most of the variance in a set of data. [Chapter 6]

Probability (*p*) is a measure of the uncertainty of the occurrence of an event, such that a probability of 0 means that an event cannot happen and a probability of 1 means it is bound to happen. It may be expressed as a decimal (e.g. 0.05, 0.01), percentage (e.g. 5%, 1%) or proportion (e.g. 1 in 20, 1:20, 1 in 100, 1:100). [Chapter 9]

Psychometric properties: the validity and reliability of a measure. [Chapter 6]

Quartile: The value that demarks the highest or lowest 25% of the sample or population. [Chapter 6]

Random sample: sample selected using a random process and is representative of the population from which it is drawn. [Chapter 7]

Range is an indication of the spread of values, and is given by the highest and lowest measurements recorded. [Chapters 5, 6]

Rank refers to position in the hierarchy when all measurements are set out from lowest to highest. Data are converted to ranks for analysis if they are ordinal, or if they are interval but do not conform to the normal distribution. [Chapter 6]

Raw data: data in the form in which they were originally collected.

Regression (linear regression) is used to predict the value of a single interval dependent (outcome) variable, using one or more independent (predictor) variables.

- *Simple linear regression* is used if there is one interval independent variable and one interval dependent variable, and both conform to the normal distribution. [Chapter 15]

- *Multiple regression* is used if the dependent variable is interval. [Chapter 16]

- *Logistic regression* is used if the dependent variable consists of two categories. [Chapter 16]

Regression to the mean: a natural tendency for average measurements or individual test scores (including depression) to drift towards the population average over time.

Relative risk (RR) is a measure of the risk or benefit in one condition, compared to the risk or benefit in another condition.

Reliability: A reliable measure is one that consistently gives the same measurement when used in the same conditions. [Chapter 4]

- *Test–reliability* measures the extent to which the measure gives the same results on different occasions under the same conditions.
- *Split-half reliability* determines if two similar sets of items give the same results.
- *Inter-rater reliability* is used to measure the extent to which two independent observers record the same result when observing the same event or phenomenon.

Representative sample refers to a sample that shares the same characteristics as the population from which it is taken. [Chapter 7]

Rotation: used in factor analysis to maximise the differentiation between common factors (Chapter 6). The most common procedures are:

- *Varimax rotation* assumes that the factors are unrelated to each other (orthogonal)
- *Oblique rotation* is used if the factors are not entirely independent of each other.

Scatterplot or scatter diagram is a graph of the values of one interval variable plotted against the values of a second interval variable. It is used to check if the relationship is linear and to identify 'outliers'. [Chapter 11]

Sign test: Similar to the Wilcoxon test; used to determine if two paired measurements are significantly different. [Chapter 13]

Significance level (level of alpha): the level of probability (p value) at which the results are confirmed as statistically significant: i.e. the null hypothesis is rejected and the researcher's hypothesis is supported. [Chapter 9]

Skewed / skewness refers to data that tend to cluster towards one end of the distribution (range of measurements). [Chapter 5]

SPSS Statistical Package for the Social Sciences. Probably the most common computer package used to analyse statistical data.

Spearman's rho (r_s): a test of correlation used where the data are ordinal or for interval data with a non-normal distribution. [Chapter 15]

Standard deviation (sd) is a standardised measure of spread or variation in the data, assuming that the data conform to the pattern of the normal distribution. It measures the distance from the mean in the units in which the data were originally measured. [Chapter 5]

Standard error of the mean (SEM) is a measure of the predicted variability of the sample mean. It has largely been replaced by the use of the confidence interval (CI) which is easier to interpret.

Statistical significance implies that the researcher's hypothesis is true and there is a difference between groups or a relationship between variables. [Chapter 9]

Stratified random sampling is used when two or more comparison groups within a population (e.g. males and females) are present in grossly unequal numbers. [Chapter 7]

Type I (one) error refers to a false positive or spurious result. The researcher's hypothesis is held to be true when there really is no difference or association. [Chapter 9]

Type II (two) error refers to a false negative result. The researcher's hypothesis is rejected when it is actually true. [Chapter 9]

Validity: A valid measure is one that accurately represents the concept or construct that it is intended to measure. [Chapter 6]

- *Face validity*: does it look right at face value?
- *Content validity*: are all aspects of relevant content present and no important aspects missing?
- *Construct validity*: is the measure conceptually coherent?
- *Predictive validity*: does the measure accurately predict verifiable outcomes or consequences?
- *Concurrent validity*: does the measure give similar results to previously validated measures?

Value: refers to a recorded measurement.

Variable refers to a measurable condition or characteristic that reflects difference in group membership (e.g. ethnic origin) or is amenable to change.

Variance: in statistics, this is a measure of the spread or distribution of the data. In numerical terms, it is equal to the square of the standard deviation.

Variance Inflation Factor (VIF): test used to identify multicollinearity prior to multiple regression analysis.

Zero-order correlation: the correlation between 2 variables.

III Guide to Statistical Symbols

Signifiers

= equal to

< less than

≤ less than or equal to

> more than

≥ more than or equal to

± plus or minus

Symbols used to signify statistical terms

α **alpha.** Significance level (level of alpha) or coefficient alpha (Cronbach's alpha).

CI   **Confidence interval.** The range of values that can be predicted with reasonable (usually 95% or 99%) certainty.

df   **Degrees of freedom.** This refers to the number of cases (n) or categories included in a statistical analysis, but also includes a small correction used to reduce the likelihood of Type I (false positive) error in the results of statistical tests, particularly where the sample size is small.
       In general:

- $df = n - 1$ where the dependent variable is interval or ordinal
- $df = (rows - 1) \times (columns - 1)$ where the data are categorical, as in contingency analysis (χ^2).

N or *n*   **Sample size,** specifically the number of cases included in the data analysis.

p   **Probability.** This is given as a number, in decimals, between 0 and 1. The value of p denotes the probability that the null hypothesis is true and there really is no difference of association in the data. [Chapter 9]
       $p \leq 0.05$ is the minimum standard for a statistically significant result, implying that there is difference between groups or relationship between variables.
       $p = 0.05$ means a probability of 5:100 or 5% or 1 in 20.
       The smaller the value of p (more noughts after the decimal point), the greater the likelihood that the results are statistically significant.

sd   **Standard deviation.** A standardised measure of the distance from the mean, based on the normal distribution. Standard deviation units are related directly to the value of p.

SE   **Standard error**: a measure of variability which is added to or subtracted from the mean, or other statistical value, to give the range of values which are reasonably certain. This has largely been replaced by the confidence interval (CI) which is easier to interpret.

SEM   **Standard error of the mean.** See standard error.

Common statistical test symbols

B   Weighting given to each independent variable in the regression equation.

β   Beta. Standardised weighting for each independent variable in multiple regression, a measure of relative importance.

F   Analysis of variance (ANOVA) or analysis of covariance (ANCOVA).

F_r Friedman ANOVA by ranks.

H or *KW*   Kruskal–Wallis test.

r   Pearson product-moment correlation coefficient.

r_s Spearman's rho correlation.

R   Regression coefficient.

R^2 Proportion of variance explained by regression model.

t   *t* test (Student's *t* test).

τ   Kendall's tau.

U   Mann–Whitney *U* test.

Φ   Phi correlation.

χ^2 Chi-square.

W   Wilcoxon signed rank test.

z score   Standard deviation units.

IV Overview of Common Statistical Tests

Tests of group difference

Tests of group difference (see Chapters 11–14) are used to compare two or more independent (unrelated) groups.

The reviewer must check that the assumptions of each statistical test have been met. These include:

- the number of groups to be compared;
- the type and distribution of the dependent (comparison) variable;
- the presence of repeated measures or matched samples.

Analysis of variance (ANOVA) and **analysis of covariance (ANCOVA)**, and the associated **F test**, are parametric tests used if the dependent (outcome) variable is interval and conforms to the normal distribution (Chapters 12 and 14).

- **One-way ANOVA** is similar to the independent *t* test, but is used to measure the difference between the means of three or more groups.
- **ANCOVA** is similar to repeated measures ANOVA, but controls for demographic or baseline variables that might otherwise confound the findings.

Chi-square (χ^2) is used in **contingency analysis** to identify deviations from the expected distribution where both the dependent and independent variables consist of independent (unrelated) categories (Chapter 11).

Friedman test or Friedman ANOVA by ranks is the nonparametric equivalent of repeated measures ANOVA, based on rank scores (Chapter 14). The results are often given using the χ^2 **(chi-square)** test statistic.

Fisher's exact test (Fisher's exact probability) is used to compare two separate groups, where the dependent (comparison) variable has only two mutually exclusive categories. There is no test statistic as the exact probability (*p* value) is calculated directly.

Kruskal–Wallis test (*H* or *KW*) is the nonparametric equivalent of one-way ANOVA. It is used to compare three or more separate groups, based on rank scores (Chapter 12). The results are often given using the χ^2 **(chi-square)** statistic.

Multivariate analysis of variance (MANOVA) is similar to ANOVA, but there is more than one dependent (outcome) variable.

***t* test (Student's *t* test)** is used to compare two groups where the dependent variable is interval and conforms to the normal distribution (Chapter 11).

- The **unrelated (independent)** *t* **test** is used to compare the same measurements taken from two separate groups.
- The **related (paired)** *t* **test** is used to compare the same measurements taken from the same group at different points in time, or from matched individuals.

Mann–Whitney *U* **test** is the nonparametric equivalent of the unrelated *t* test. It is used to compare two separate groups based on rank scores (Chapter 11). The results for samples greater than 20 are given as a *z* **score**.

Wilcoxon test / signed rank test is the nonparametric equivalent of the related (paired) *t* test. It is used to compare repeated measurements from a single sample, or data from matched samples, using rank scores (Chapter 13). Results for samples greater than 20 are given as a *z* **score**.

z **score** is interpreted as **standard deviation units** and relates directly to the position on the normal distribution curve.

Based on the normal distribution, a two-tailed *z* score of 2 or greater (2 or more standard deviations from the mean) will give a *p* value less than 0.05 (Chapter 4).

Similarly, a two-tailed *z* score of 3 or greater will give a *p* value less than 0.01.

z **score** is often given as the result of a nonparametric test of group difference. It is a standardised difference score that is interpreted in terms of probability, as above.

Post hoc tests of multiple comparison

These are used to test for difference between each pair of variables following a significant result using ANOVA or ANCOVA (see Chapters 12 and 14). They include:

- **Tukey's HSD** (honestly significant difference);
- **Scheffé test**;
- **Least significant difference test**, equivalent to doing multiple pairwise *t* tests.

Tests of association

Tests of association are used to test the strength of relationships between two or more variables.

The reviewer must check that the assumptions of each statistical test have been met. These include:

- the type and distribution of the dependent (outcome) variable;
- the relationship between the variables must be linear (follow a straight line);
- where there is more than one independent (predictor) variable, these should not be closely correlated.

Correlation

Pearson product-moment correlation coefficient (*r*) is a parametric test of association used for continuous variables that approximate to the normal distribution (Chapter 15).

Spearman's rho (r_s) is the nonparametric equivalent of the Pearson product-moment correlation, calculated using rank values rather than actual values. It is a nonparametric test used for ordinal data and interval data that are skewed (Chapter 15).

Phi (Φ) is a test of correlation used when both variables are dichotomous.

Kendall's tau (τ) is a nonparametric test of correlation, used as an alternative to Spearman's rho.

Regression

R Printed as a capital letter, R is the **regression coefficient**. This is a number between 0 and 1 (or 0 and −1) which is interpreted in the same way as the correlation coefficient (Chapter 15).

R^2 The square of the R value is a more realistic measure of association in multiple regression analysis. It is usually given as a percentage which measures the extent to which the combined set of independent (predictor) variables explain the dependent (outcome) variable (Chapter 16).

B In multiple regression, B is the weighting given to each independent (predictor) variable in order to predict the value of the dependent (outcome variable (Y) from the regression equation:

$$Y = B_1X_1 + B_2X_2 + \ldots + (constant)$$

where X_1, X_2 etc. are the values for each of the independent variables.

β In multiple regression, **beta** is the standardised weighting that measures the relative importance of each of the independent variable.

Other statistical tests

There are many other statistical tests that are not included in this book. In case you encounter these, we give a brief overview of some of them.

Tests for skewness

Data exhibiting skewness tend to cluster towards one end of the distribution (range of measurements).

Pearson's skewness coefficient is a simple measure of skewness given by

$$\frac{\text{mean} - \text{median}}{\text{standard deviation}}.$$

A value of 0 indicates a normal distribution. Values greater than 0.2 or less than −0.2 indicate a skewed distribution.

Fisher's measure of skewness uses a computer-based calculation. Values greater than 1.96 or less than −1.96 indicate a significantly skewed distribution.

Tests for kurtosis

Kurtosis describes a data distribution that is too flat or peaked to analyse using parametric statistics that rely on assumptions of normal distribution.

Fisher's measure of kurtosis uses a computer-based calculation. Values greater than 1.96 indicate the curve is likely to be too peaked to analyse using parametric statistics, while values less than –1.96 indicate that the curve is likely to be too flat.

Tests for homogeneity of variance

These tests are applied where two or more groups or samples are to be compared. It tests if the distributions of the data are approximately the same for each group. This is a requirement for the t test and ANOVA.

Box's M is used in analysis of variance to ensure that the data taken from separate (independent) groups have equal variances or standard deviations. A statistically significant result indicates that the normal distribution is violated. However, the test is extremely sensitive and may overestimate the importance of differences in variance. Tabachnik and Fidell (1989) suggested that homogeneity of variance could not be guaranteed if $p < 0.001$, especially if the sample sizes are unequal.

Tests of sphericity

The inverted U-shaped curve reflects the normal distribution for a single variable. In multivariate analysis, where variables are combined, the shape is spherical (like a round ball). In all cases, the distribution should be symmetrical in order to meet the requirements of parametric tests that rely on the normal distribution. 'Odd' shaped distributions are likely to lead to unreliable results.

Maunchley's test is used in repeated measures analysis of variance to ensure that the data demonstrate compound symmetry. A value of $p \leq 0.05$ indicates that the assumption is violated.

Goodness-of-fit tests

These tests are used to measure the extent to which the variance included in a statistical model adequately explains the total variance in the data set.

Chi-square (χ^2) test is most commonly used. A non-significant result indicates no difference between the model and the data. Therefore, $p \leq 0.05$ indicates a poor fit.

Bartlett's test is used in factor analysis to assess the overall strength of correlation between included variables. This test is extremely sensitive and although $p < 0.05$ is significant, smaller values of p are more desirable.

Factor analysis/principle components analysis

Factor analysis and principle components analysis are used to group a large number of items into a smaller number of factors or concepts, or to confirm the construct validity of a measurement scale.

Procedures used in factor analysis include:

1. The method of factor extraction. Popular methods include:
   - **Principle components analysis** (accounts for all variance);
   - **Maximum likelihood**;
   - **Unweighted least squares**.
2. The method of rotation. Rotation is used to improve interpretation of the emergent factors.
   - **Orthogonal rotation** assumes that each factor is independent of each other factor. The most popular procedure is varimax rotation.
   - **Oblique rotation** is used when there is considerable overlap between emergent factors. It is used to maximise separation. The most common procedure is oblimin rotation.

Statistics associated with the stages and results of factor analysis include the following:

1. **Eigenvalues** measure the amount of variance explained by each factor. Usually, an eigenvalue greater than 1 is required for a factor to be considered as unique in factor analysis.
2. **Percentage variance** is the percentage of the total variance in the data that is explained by each emergent factor.
3. **Communality** measures the contribution of each item to the emergent factor model in factor analysis. (Communality in principle components analysis is 1.00 because each item is treated as a separate factor.)
4. **Factor scores** are standardised measures that represent the relative contribution of each item to each emergent factor in factor analysis.
5. **Tests of validity and reliability** [Chapter 6]
6. **Cronbach's alpha** measure of internal consistency on a scale of 0 to 1: >0.8 is good; >0.6 is acceptable.
7. **Kappa** measure of inter-rater agreement: >0.8 is very good; >0.6 is good.
8. **Bland-Altman plot** used to measure inter-rater agreement. Bias is judged by the proportion of values that fall either above or below the 95% confidence interval.

V Guide to the Assumptions that Underpin Statistical Tests

The onus is on the researchers to ensure that these assumptions were met if they have used these tests, and on the reviewer to check that they have done this.

Tests of group difference

Parametric tests

Independent *t* test and one-way ANOVA (*F* test):

- The groups are independent (unrelated).
- The dependent variable is measured using a continuous scale, normally with at least 11 points and equal intervals (Chapter 3).
- These data approximate to the normal distribution (Chapter 4).
- The standard deviations for each group are approximately the same (this is termed 'homogeneity of variance').

Related *t* test for matched pairs or repeated measures and repeated measures ANOVA or ANCOVA (*F* test):

- Data for each group are related – either matched pairs or repeated measures.
- The dependent variable is measured using a continuous scale, normally with at least 11 points and equal intervals (Chapter 3).
- The data approximate to the normal distribution (Chapter 4).

Nonparametric tests

Mann–Whitney *U* test and Kruskal–Wallis one-way ANOVA by ranks:

- The groups are independent (unrelated).
- The dependent variable is measured using an ordinal or continuous scale that has at least 4 points on the scale (Chapter 3).

Wilcoxon test, signed rank test and Friedman two-way ANOVA by ranks:

- Data for each group are related, either using matched pairs or repeated measures.
- The dependent variable is measured using a continuous or ordinal scale that has at least four points on the scale (Chapter 3).

Contingency analysis (categorical data)

Fisher exact test and chi-square test:

- The data are based on frequency counts.
- There are no related data (no matched pairs or repeated measures).
- Each observation is recorded in only one category (cell).

Tests of correlation

Pearson product-moment correlation (r):

- Both variables are taken from the same sample, or from matched pairs.
- Both variables are measured using a continuous scale.
- The data approximate to the normal distribution and are spread across the full range of the scale.
- The relationship between the two variables is linear.
- Correlation between the two variables does not imply there is a causal relationship.

Spearman rank correlation (Spearman's rho, r_s) and Kendall's tau

- Both variables are taken from the same sample, or from matched pairs
- Both variables are measured using a scale that has at least 4 data points
- The data are spread across the full range of the scale.
- The relationship between the two variables is linear.
- Correlation between the two variables does not imply there is a causal relationship.

Regression

Simple linear regression (R):

- Both variables are taken from the same sample, or from matched pairs.
- Both variables are measured using a continuous scale.
- The data approximate to the normal distribution and are spread across the full range of the scale.
- The relationship between the independent variables is linear.
- There is sound theoretical reason to predict a causal relationship between the independent (predictor) variable and the dependent (outcome) variable.

Multiple regression:

- There is sound theoretical justification for predicting that the dependent (outcome) variable will be predicted by a combination of the independent (predictor) variables.

- The relationship between the independent variables and the dependent variable is linear.
- The dependent variable is measured using a continuous scale and approximates to the normal distribution.
- The independent variables are either continuous and conform to the normal distribution, or may be dichotomous.
- There is no evidence of multicollinearity between the independent variables – this means that the independent variables are not closely correlated.
- The regression model should demonstrate homoscedascity – the variation around the regression line is the same for all values of each independent variable.

Logistic regression:

- The dependent variable is dichotomous.
- The independent variable may be measured using any level of measurement from categorical to continuous.

VI Summary of Statistical Test Selection and Results

Descriptive statistics (Chapters 4 and 5)

Measurement	Parametric data	Nonparametric data	Categorical data
	Continuous, interval data (11+ data points) Normal distribution	*Ordinal (4+ data points) Non-normal distribution*	*Discrete (independent) categories*
Central tendency	Mean	Median	Percentages
Distribution (spread)	Standard deviation (sd) Variance (= sd^2)	Percentiles Interquartile range	
Range	Minimum/maximum value	Minimum/maximum value	
Visual presentation	Histogram	Bar chart	Bar chart/pie chart

Test of normal distribution

- The mean is in the middle of the range.
- The mean is equal to the median.
- The distribution is somewhat skewed if (mean ± 2 standard deviations) lies outside actual or possible range.
- The distribution is very skewed if (mean ± 1 standard deviation) lies outside the actual or possible range.

Inferential statistics

Tests of comparison (Chapters 11 and 12)

Number of groups or measures	Parametric tests	Nonparametric tests	Categorical data
	Continuous data Normal distribution Equal group variances n ≥ 30	*Ordinal data Non-normal distribution n < 30*	*Independent categories*
Between-group comparisons			
2 groups	Unrelated *t* test	Mann–Whitney *U* test	Fisher exact test (2 × 2 table)
>2 groups	One-way ANOVA (*F* test)	Kruskal–Wallis ANOVA by rank	Chi-square test (χ^2)
Within-group comparisons (repeated measures)			
2 measures	Related *t* test	Wilcoxon signed rank test	McNemar change test
>2 measures	Two-way (repeated measures) ANOVA	Friedman two-way ANOVA by rank	
Between groups and repeated measures			
	Factorial ANOVA		

Tests of association (Chapters 15 and 16)

Parametric tests	Nonparametric tests	Categorical data
Continuous data Normal distribution $n \geq 30$	Ordinal data Non-normal distribution	Independent categories
Correlation between 2 variables		
Pearson product-moment correlation (r)	Spearman's rho (r_s) Kendall's rank correlation	Cramer coefficient Phi (r_ϕ)
Partial correlation (controls for effect of a third variable)		
Regression: 2 variables		
Simple regression		
Regression: 1 dependent (outcome) variable, 2+ independent (predictor) variables		
Multiple regression	Logistic regression	

Results of correlation

- **Test statistic:** r, r_s, r_ϕ; r is a number between 0 and 1, interpreted in social science contexts as follows:

  0–0.15 = no association

  0.15–0.29 = weak association

  0.3–0.59 = moderate association

  0.6+ strong association
- n: number of cases/respondents, or **df** $(n - 2)$
- p: probability that there is *no* association between the variables

Results of regression analysis

- **B**: weighting for each variable in the regression equation

  $$Y = B_1 X_1 + B_2 X_2 \ldots + A$$

  where Y is the value of the dependent (outcome)variable;
  X_1, X_2 etc. are the values for each of independent (predictor) variables;
  B_1, B_2, etc. are the weightings for each independent variable; and A is the value of a constant that allows for unknown independent variables and error
- β **(beta)**: a measure of the relative importance of each independent variable as a predictor
- p: probability that the independent variable does *not* make a significant contribution to the regression model

- **R**: the regression coefficient, interpreted as for correlation (*r*)
- **R²**: the proportion of variance explained by the regression model – this represents the explanatory power of the result.

Other statistics are used, but these are most important. Researchers normally give *B* or *β*, but not necessarily both.

Treatment outcomes (Chapter 16)

Relative risk (RR)

$$RR = \frac{\text{proportion in group A with outcome } Y}{\text{proportion in group B with outcome } Y}$$

Odds ratio (OR)

$$OR = \frac{\text{probability of occurrence/probability of non-occurrence (group A)}}{\text{probability of occurrence/probability of non-occurrence (group B)}}$$

Number needed to treat (NNT) refers to the number of people who need to receive treatment in order for one person to benefit (for formula, see Chapter 16).

Tests of validity and reliability (Chapter 6)

Coefficient alpha (Cronbach's alpha or *α*)
Test–retest reliability
Inter-rater reliability

Each of these is measured on a scale of 0 to 1:

0.8+	Good
0.7–0.79	Acceptable
0.6–0.69	Weak
less than 0.6	Unacceptable

VII Extracts from Statistical Tables

The following tables give 'critical values' for some common statistical tests. The values given are intended as a rough guide for reviewers and are approximated to one or two decimal places.

We have assumed that df (degrees of freedom) approximates to the value of n (the number of complete sets of data included in the analysis). These figures are not intended for use by researchers.

Values for the test statistic are given in the shaded area of each table. The test statistic must be greater than or equal to the critical value given in order to achieve significance at the value of p given.

Pearson correlation coefficient: critical values of r

	Directional (one-tailed) p				
	0.05	0.025	0.01	0.005	0.0005
n	Non-directional (two-tailed) p				
	0.1	0.05	0.02	0.01	0.001
20	0.36	0.42	0.49	0.54	0.65
30	0.30	0.35	0.41	0.45	0.55
50	0.23	0.27	0.32	0.35	0.44
80	0.18	0.22	0.26	0.28	0.36
100	0.16	0.19	0.23	0.25	0.32

Example

Suppose that $r = 0.43$ and $n = 35$. Find the closest approximation to n in the left-hand column (i.e. $n = 30$) and follow the horizontal numbers to find the largest value of r less than or equal to 0.43 (i.e. 0.41). Now read up the column to find the value of p. This gives the following conservative approximations: $p < 0.02$ (two-tailed) and $p < 0.01$ (one-tailed).

t test: critical values of *t*

df	Directional (one-tailed) *p*				
	0.05	0.025	0.01	0.005	0.0005
	Non-directional (two-tailed) *p*				
	0.1	0.05	0.02	0.01	0.001
20	1.7	2.1	2.5	2.8	3.9
30	1.7	2.0	2.5	2.8	3.6
60	1.7	2.0	2.4	2.7	3.5
120+	1.6	2.0	2.3	2.6	3.3

Suppose that the difference between the group means is 5.1, and the standard deviation across both groups is 1.8. Then $t = 5.1/1.8 = 2.8$. If $n = 168$ (df = 166), then the value of *p* will be $p < 0.01$ (two-tailed) and $p < 0.005$ (one-tailed).

Example

Chi-square: critical values of χ^2

df*	Directional (one-tailed) p				
	0.05	0.025	0.01	0.005	0.0005
	Non-directional (two-tailed) p				
	0.1	0.05	0.02	0.01	0.001
1	2.7	3.8	5.4	6.6	10.8
2	4.6	6.0	7.8	9.2	13.8
6	10.6	12.6	15.0	16.8	22.5
10	16.0	18.3	21.2	23.2	30.0

*df = (rows − 1) × (columns − 1)

Suppose that the table consists of 3 rows and 4 columns. Then df = (3 − 1) × (4 − 1) = 6. If $\chi^2 = 11.3$, then the value of *p* will be $p > 0.05$ (two-tailed) and $p < 0.05$ (one-tailed). The two-tailed test gives a non-significant result.

Example

ANOVA: Critical values of *F*
$p = 0.05$ (plain text); $p = 0.01$ (bold text).

df (groups–1)	df (n-groups)					
	20	30	40	50	100	1000
1	4.4	4.2	4.1	4.0	3.9	3.9
	8.1	**7.6**	**7.3**	**7.2**	**6.9**	**6.6**
2	3.5	3.3	3.2	3.2	3.1	3.0
	5.8	**5.4**	**5.2**	**5.1**	**4.8**	**4.6**

Note that one-tailed and two-tailed tests of significance are not differentiated in standard statistical tables, but can be differentiated in computerised versions.

Example

Suppose that $F(1, 59) = 6.3$. This implies that ANOVA was used to compare 2 groups, with a complete set of data from a sample of $n = 60$. The value of p will be $p < 0.05$.

References

Achenbach, T. (2008) *Child Behavior Checklist for Ages 6–18 (CBCL/6–18)* http://www.aseba.org/products/cbcl6-18.html (accessed 12 October 2008).

Altman, D.G. and Bland, J.M. (1983) Measurement in medicine: the analysis of method comparison studies. *The Statistician*, 32: 307–317.

Atherton, K., Fuller, E., Shepherd, P., Strachan, D.P. and Power, C. (2008) Loss and representativeness in a biomedical survey at age 45 years: 1958 British birth cohort. *Journal of Epidemiology & Community Health*, 62: 216–223.

Bandolier (1996) *Swots corner: what's an odds ratio?* http://www.medicine.ox.ac.uk/bandolier/band25/b25-6.html (accessed 9 November 2008).

Bartlett, J.E., Kotrlik, J.W. and Higgins, C.C. (2001) Organizational research: determining appropriate sample size in survey research. *Information Technology, Learning, and Performance Journal*, 19: 43–50.

Berry, D., Courtenay, M. and Bersellini, E. (2006) Attitudes towards, and information needs in relation to, supplementary nurse prescribing in the UK: an empirical study. *Journal of Clinical Nursing*, 15: 22–28.

Bowling, A. (2005) *Measuring Health*, 3rd edition. Maidenhead: Open University Press.

Broll, S., Glaser, S. and Kreienbrock, L. (2002) Calculating sample size bounds for logistic regression. *Preventive Veterinary Medicine*, 54: 105–111.

Chisholm, V., Atkinson, L., Donaldson, C., Noyes, K., Payne, A. and Kelnar, C. (2007) Predictors of treatment adherence in young children with type 1 diabetes. *Journal of Advanced Nursing*, 57(5): 482–493.

Claesson, I., Sydsjö, G., Brynhildsen, J., Cedergren, M., Jeppsson, A., Nyström, F., Sydsjö, A. and Josefsson, A. (2007) Weight gain restriction for obese pregnant women: a case–control intervention study. *British Journal of Obstetrics and Gynaecology*, 115: 44–50.

Coe, R. (2000) *What is an 'effect size'? A brief introduction.* http://www.cemcentre.org/renderpage.asp?linkid=30325016 (accessed 16 November 2008).

Cohen, J. (1988) *Statistical Power Analysis for the Behavioral Sciences*, 2nd edition. Hillsdale, NJ: Lawrence Erlbaum Associates.

Dancey, C.P. and Reidy, J. (2007) *Statistics without Maths for Psychology: Using SPSS for Windows*, 4th edition. London: Pearson Prentice Hall.

Fallis, D. and Fricke, M. (2002) Indicators of accuracy of consumer health information on the internet. *Journal of the American Medical Informatics Association*, 9: 73–79.

Field, A. (2009) *Discovering Statistics Using SPSS*, 3rd edition. London: Sage.

Gilbertson, L., Langhorne, P., Walker, A., Allen, A. and Murray, G.D. (2000) Domiciliary occupational therapy for patients with stroke discharged from hospital: randomised controlled trial. *British Medical Journal*, 320(7235): 603–606.

Graff, M.J.L., Vernooij-Dassen, M.J.M., Thijssen, M., Dekker, J., Hoefnagels, W.H.L. and Rikkert, M.G.M.O. (2006) Community based occupational therapy for patients with dementia and their care givers: randomised controlled trial. *British Medical Journal*, 333: 1196.

Hagell, P., Törnqvist, A.L. and Hobart, J. (2008) Testing the SF-36 in Parkinson's disease. Implications for reporting rating scale data. *Journal of Neurology*, 255: 246–254.

Hagen, L.E.M., Schneider, R., Stephens, D., Modrusan, D. and Feldman, B.M. (2003) Use of complementary and alternative medicine by pediatric rheumatology patients. *Arthritis & Rheumatism*, 49: 3–6.

Harwood, R.H. and Ebrahim, S. (2002) The validity, reliability and responsiveness of the Nottingham Extended Activities of Daily Living scale in patients undergoing total hip replacement. *Disability and Rehabilitation*, 24(7): 371–377.

Holland, R., Lenaghan, E., Harvey, I., Smith, R., Shepstone, L., Lipp, A., Christou, M., Evans, D. and Hand, C. (2005). Does home based medication review keep older people out of hospital? The HOMER randomised controlled trial. *British Medical Journal*, 330: 293.

Ilhan, M.N., Durukan, E., Taner, E., Maral, I. and Bumin, M.A. (2008) Burnout and its correlates among nursing staff: questionnaire survey. *Journal of Advanced Nursing*, 61: 100–106.

Jaeger, R.M. (1983) *Statistics: Spectator Sport*, 2nd edition. Newbury Park, CA: Sage.

Janssen, I., Katzmarzyk, P.T. and Ross, R. (2004) Waist circumference and not body mass index explains obesity-related health risk. *American Journal of Clinical Nutrition*, 79: 379–384.

Jebb, S.A., Rennie, K.L. and Cole, T.J. (2003) Prevalence of overweight and obesity among young people in Great Britain. *Public Health Nutrition*, 7: 461–465.

Jellesma, F.C., Rieffe, C. and Terwogt, M.M. (2008) My peers, my friend, and I: Peer interactions and somatic complaints in boys and girls. *Social Science & Medicine*, 66: 2195–2205.

Johansson, S., Ytterberg, C., Hillert, J., Holmqvist, W. and von Koch, L. (2008) A longitudinal study of variations in and predictors of fatigue in multiple sclerosis. *Journal of Neurological and Neurosurgical Psychiatry*, 79: 454–457.

Johnson, S.B., Silverstein, J., Rosenbloom, A., Carter, R. and Cunningham, W. (1986) Assessing daily management in childhood diabetes. *Health Psychology*, 5: 545–564.

Keeley, P., Creed, F., Tomenson, B., Todd, C., Borglin, G. and Dickens, C. (2008) Psychosocial predictors of health-related quality of life and health service utilisation in people with chronic low back pain. *Pain*, 135: 142–150.

Kovacs, F.M., Abraira, V., Zamora, J., del Real, M.T.G., Llobera, J. and Carmen Fernandez, C. (2004) Correlation between pain, disability, and quality of life in patients with common low back pain. *Spine*, 29: 206–210.

Landis, J.R. and Koch, G.G. (1977) The measurement of observer agreement for categorical data. *Biometrics*, 33: 159–174.

Logan, P.A., Gladman, J.R.F., Avery, A., Walker, M.F., Dyas, J. and Groom, L. (2004) Randomised controlled trial of an occupational therapy intervention to increase outdoor mobility after stroke. *British Medical Journal*, 329: 1372–1375.

Magnussen, P.K.E., Rasmussen, F. and Gyllensten, U.D. (2006) Height at age 18 years is a strong predictor of attained education later in life: cohort study of over 950 000 Swedish men. *International Journal of Epidemiology*, 35: 658–663.

Mangunkusumo, R.T., Brug, J., Duisterhout, J.S., de Koning, H.J. and Raat, H. (2007) Feasibility, acceptability, and quality of internet-administered adolescent health promotion in a preventive-care setting. *Health Education Research*, 22: 1–13.

McHorney, C.A. and Tarlov, A.R. (1995) Individual-patient monitoring in clinical practice: are available health status surveys adequate? *Quality of Life Research*, 4: 293–307.

Nishimura, R., Tsujino, D., Taki, K., Morimoto, A., Tajima, N. and Nishimura, R. (2008) Does HbA1c represent a valid index for tight control of glucose in type 1 diabetes? *Diabetes Research and Clinical Practice*, 82: e23–e24.

Pare, P., Ferrazzi, S., Thompson, W.G., Irvine, E.J., Rance, L. (2001) An epidemiological survey of constipation in Canada: definitions, rates, demographics, and predictors of health care seeking. *American Journal of Gastroenterology*, 96: 3130–3137.

Pett, M.A. (1997) *Nonparametric Statistics for Health Care Research: Statistics for Small Samples and Unusual Distributions*. Thousand Oaks, CA: Sage.

Pincus, T. and Wolfe, F. (2005) Patient questionnaires for clinical research and improved standard patient care: is it better to have 80% of the information in 100% of patients or 100% of the information in 5% of patients? *Journal of Rheumatology*, 32: 575–577.

Redmond, A.C. and Keenan, A.-M. (2002) Understanding statistics: putting *p*-values into perspective. *Journal of the American Podiatric Medical Association*, 92: 297–305.

Richards, D.A., Lovell, K., Gilbody, S., Gask, L., Torgerson, D., Barkham, M. and Bland, M. (2008) Collaborative care for depression in UK primary care: a randomized controlled trial. *Psychological Medicine*, 38: 279–287.

Siegel, S. and Castellan, N.J. (1988) *Nonparametric Statistics for the Behavioral Sciences*, 2nd edition. New York, McGraw-Hill.

Tabachnik, B.G. and Fidell, L.S. (1989) *Using Multivariate Statistics*, 2nd edition. New York: Harper & Row.

Thurston, R.C., Sowers, M.R., Chang, Y., Sternfeld, B., Gold, E.B., Johnston, J.M. and Matthews, K.A. (2007) Adiposity and reporting of vasomotor symptoms among midlife women: The Study of Women's Health Across the Nation. *American Journal of Epidemiology*, 167: 78–85.

Torgerson, D.J., Campbell, M.K., Reid, D.M. (1995) Life-style, environmental and medical factors influencing peak bone mass in women. *British Journal of Rheumatology*, 34: 620–624.

Index

The index entries appear in word-by-word alphabetical order.

A BEGINNER'S GUIDE TO EVIDENCE-BASED PRACTICE IN HEALTH AND SOCIAL CARE

Helen Aveyard; Pam Sharp

"I would just like to say this is the best text I have come across for my module for under-graduate students. It is pitched at just the right level and is written in a style that is easy to engage with. The layout and the structure are also easy to follow and it is a really good introduction to EBP. I intend recommending this to my students and thank you once again for sending me a copy of this."

Jean Davison, Teesside University, UK

Have you heard of 'evidence based practice' but don't know what it means? Are you having trouble relating evidence to your practice?

This is the book for anyone who has ever wondered what evidence based practice is or how to relate it to practice. This accessible book presents the topic in a simple, easy to understand way, enabling those unfamiliar with evidence based practice to apply the concept to their practice and learning.

Using everyday language, this book provides a step by step guide to what we mean by evidence based practice and how to apply it. It also:

- Provides an easy to follow guide to searching for evidence
- Explains how to work out if the evidence is relevant or not
- Explores how evidence can be applied in the practice setting
- Outlines how evidence can be incorporated into your academic writing

A Beginner's Guide to Evidence Based Practice in Health and Social Care is key reading for everyone involved in looking at and applying evidence - students, practice educators, mentors and practising health and social care professionals.

Contents: *Acknowledgements - Introduction - What is evidence based practice? - The development of evidence based practice When do we need to use evidence and what evidence do we need? - What are the different types of research? - How do I find the evidence to support my practice and learning? - How do I know if the evidence is convincing and useful? - How to use and implement evidence in your practice and learning - References - Appendix A - Glossary - Appendix B Useful Web Links*

2009 224pp
978-0-335- 23603-9 (Paperback)   978-0-335- 23602-2 (Hardback)

RESEARCH METHODS IN HEALTH 3/e
Ann Bowling

This bestselling book provides an accessible introduction to the theoretical concepts and descriptive and analytic research methods used in research on health and health services. The third edition has been thoroughly revised throughout to include updated references and boxed examples, with additional information on key methodological developments, among them:

- Complex interventions
- Mixed research methods
- Psychometrics
- Secondary data analysis
- Systematic reviews
- Pertinent social science concepts

The research methods described cover the assessment of health needs, morbidity and mortality trends and rates, costing health services, sampling for survey research, cross-sectional and longitudinal survey design, experimental methods and techniques of group assignment, questionnaire design, interviewing techniques, coding and analysis of quantitative data, methods and analysis of qualitative observational studies, and types of unstructured interviewing.

The book is grounded in the author's career as a researcher on health and health service issues, and the valuable experience this has provided in meeting the challenges of research on people and organisations in real life settings.

Research Methods in Health is an essential companion for students and researchers of health and health services, health clinicians and policy-makers with responsibility for applying research findings and judging the soundness of research.

Contents: *Evaluating health services - Social research on health: Sociological and psychological concepts and approaches - Health needs and their assessment: demography and epidemiology - Costing health services: Health economics - The philosophical framework of measurement - The principles of research - Sample size and sampling for quantitative research - Quantitative research: Surveys - Quantitative research - Sample selection and group assignment methods in experiments and other analytic methods Data collection methods in quantitative research - Questionnaire design - Techniques of survey interviewing - Preparation of quantitative data for coding and analysis - Unstructured and structured observational studies - Unstructured interviewing and focus groups - Other methods using both qualitative and quantitative approaches: Case studies, consensus methods, action research and document research – Glossary – References - Index*

2009   496pp
978-0-335-23364-9 (Paperback)